First Steps

YOUR HEALTHY LIVING JOURNAL

Active Living Partners

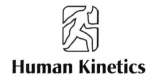

Human Kinetics

Library of Congress Cataloging-in-Publication Data

First steps : your healthy living journal.
 p. cm.
 ISBN 0-7360-6349-8 (soft cover)
 1. Exercise. 2. Nutrition. 3. Self-care, Health. 4. Self-help techniques.
 5. Diaries--Therapeutic use. I. Title: Your healthy living journal. II. Human
Kinetics.
 RA781.F545 2006
 613.7--dc22

                                          2005027056

ISBN: 0-7360-6349-8

The Web addresses cited in this text were current as of September 2005, unless otherwise noted.

Acquisitions Editor: Michele Guerra; **Managing Editor:** Wendy McLaughlin; **Assistant Editors:** Kim Thoren, Carla Zych; **Copyeditor:** Janann Feeney; **Proofreader:** Bethany J. Bentley; **Permission Manager:** Carly Breeding; **Graphic Designer:** Fred Starbird; **Graphic Artist:** Tara Welsch; **Photo Manager:** Dan Wendt; **Cover Designer:** Keith Blomberg; **Photographer (cover):** Sarah Ritz; **Art Manager:** Kareema McLendon-Foster; **Illustrator:** Human Kinetics; **Printer:** United Graphics

Human Kinetics books are available at special discounts for bulk purchase. Special editions or book excerpts can also be created to specification. For details, contact the Special Sales Manager at Human Kinetics.

Printed in the United States of America   10 9 8 7 6 5 4 3 2 1

Human Kinetics
Web site: www.HumanKinetics.com

United States: Human Kinetics
P.O. Box 5076
Champaign, IL 61825-5076
800-747-4457
e-mail: humank@hkusa.com

Canada: Human Kinetics
475 Devonshire Road Unit 100
Windsor, ON N8Y 2L5
800-465-7301 (in Canada only)
e-mail: orders@hkcanada.com

Europe: Human Kinetics
107 Bradford Road
Stanningley
Leeds LS28 6AT, United Kingdom
+44 (0) 113 255 5665
e-mail: hk@hkeurope.com

Australia: Human Kinetics
57A Price Avenue
Lower Mitcham, South Australia 5062
08 8277 1555
e-mail: liaw@hkaustralia.com

New Zealand: Human Kinetics
Division of Sports Distributors NZ Ltd.
P.O. Box 300 226 Albany
North Shore City
Auckland
0064 9 448 1207
e-mail: info@humankinetics.co.nz

CONTENTS

INTRODUCTION

*"H*abit is habit. It is not to be flung out the window by anyone, but coaxed downstairs one step at a time."

—*Mark Twain*

Welcome to *First Steps: Your Healthy Living Journal.* By opening this book, you are indicating your desire to improve your life by moving more and eating better. Our hope is that by using this book, you will take the first steps toward a healthier lifestyle.

You probably know that eating healthy foods and being physically active can improve your health and quality of life. But that knowledge alone often doesn't result in healthy actions. How many times have you said, "I know I should, but . . ."? Life's daily challenges and obligations distract us from doing the things we know will benefit us. That's where *First Steps* comes in. *First Steps: Your Healthy Living Journal* is designed to help you make simple, realistic changes in your life that will get you moving toward a healthier lifestyle. As you read the book and use the journal, you will learn ways to fit physical activity and healthy eating in your daily life, despite life's challenges.

First Steps: Your Healthy Living Journal is a different and effective approach to improving your health habits. We're not just going to tell you what to do; we're going to show you *how* to do it. At Active Living Partners we've discovered that what you really need are some special tools that help you learn *how* to trade your current behaviors for healthier ones. You'll learn how to address the underlying causes of your inactivity and unhealthy eating. And you'll learn four important principles of improving your behavior:

Step 1: Build awareness. You'll identify what good health and healthy habits mean to you, what's keeping you from getting there, and how to learn from past experiences.

Step 2: Create solutions. You'll discover simple problem-solving techniques that will enable you to overcome your barriers to physical activity and healthy eating.

Step 3: Boost confidence. We'll help you increase your sense of "I can!" You'll learn how to change your self-defeating thought patterns into empowering messages.

Step 4: Sustain commitment. You'll learn how to make physical activity and healthy eating permanent parts of your life through simple goal-setting techniques.

First Steps: Your Healthy Living Journal is divided into two parts. Part I introduces you to the four principles of improving your health habits, and it provides you with tools to help get started with each. Part II is an easy-to-use journal, where you can keep track of your physical activity, eating, goals, and other behavior change skills. Simply writing down your activities and food choices will help you to discover your current habits, set new goals, learn from mistakes, and be encouraged by your successes. Quite simply, people who keep journals are more successful than those who don't. Your journal will be a personal source of motivation and inspiration.

First Steps: Your Healthy Living Journal is your partner and coach. It will help you in the following ways:

* You will be encouraged to make positive changes in your behavior. In fact, it's much easier than you may have imagined to improve your health habits.

* You will be inspired to take the first steps to a better quality of life and better health.

* You will be equipped with the tools to take those first steps.

Ready to take your first steps? Let's get started.

Part One

❧

FOUR STEPS
TO
IMPROVING
HEALTH

Step One
~
BUILD
AWARENESS

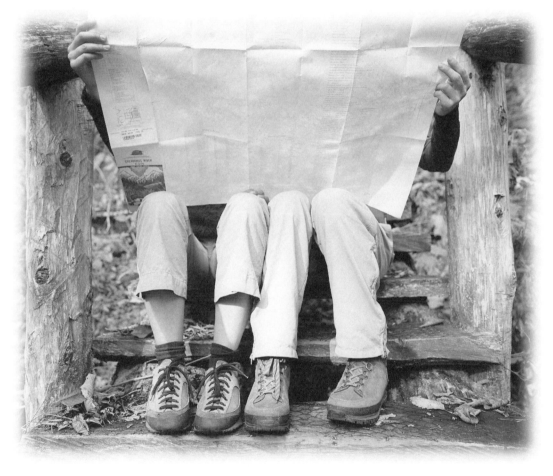

"A journey of a thousand miles begins with the first step."
—Chinese proverb

The first step to a healthy lifestyle is increasing your awareness of who you are, where you want to go, and what's holding you back. The more you know about what inspires you and what stops you from making healthy changes, the better equipped you will be to find solutions that work. Taking the time to assess these things now will give you some essential information to work with so that your future efforts will lead you to success, not just to your first roadblock.

Here are the specific areas you'll address as you build awareness that will help you improve your health habits:

* What's in it for me? Why should I change?
* Learning from my past: What's worked for me and what hasn't?
* How much is enough? What do experts say I should be doing to get enough physical activity and eat healthfully?
* What can I do to improve my health habits?

WHAT'S IN IT FOR ME?

What's been driving you to look for answers? It's simple enough to repeat what you've heard on TV or read in magazines about physical activity and healthy eating: "I want to live a longer, healthier life" or "I know that daily physical activity and healthier food choices reduce my chances of developing heart disease." But it helps to define the benefits of the healthy lifestyle in personal terms, using words and ideas that move you emotionally. For instance, if you are a grandparent, one day you may watch your grandchildren play and realize that you want to be here to see them graduate from high school 10 or 15 years from now. If you had a parent or grandparent with osteoporosis, preventing bone loss may be very important to you. You might say, "By the time my grandmother was in her 60s, she could barely stand up straight. I don't want that to happen to me." Maybe you'd simply like to have more energy. There are things you'd love to do, but you just don't have the stamina. Or perhaps you'd like to lose weight.

Healthy Habits, Great Rewards

Regular physical activity and healthy eating are essential complementary health behaviors that can help you have a better quality of life. These healthy habits will give you some or all of the following benefits:

Better weight control

More energy

Brighter mental outlook

Increased self-esteem

Reduced risk of conditions such as heart disease, cancer, high blood pressure, and diabetes

Reduced risk of colds or flu (and fewer workdays missed)

Healthy and strong bones and joints

Enhanced fitness and flexibility

Sharper mental abilities

Better quality of sleep

Increased longevity and independence later in life

FIGURE 1.1

My Benefits of Physical Activity and Healthy Eating

1._____

2._____

3._____

4._____

5._____

6._____

7._____

8._____

9._____

10._____

Take some time to identify the most important benefits of being physically active and eating more healthfully. Keeping these benefits in mind will inspire you to take action, day after day. List as many benefits as you can think of in figure 1.1. This is a very important step. Don't worry if you can think of only a couple benefits. As you learn about becoming more active and eating more healthfully, you may identify many more benefits that have meaning for you. To stimulate your thinking, read the box titled "Healthy Habits, Great Rewards," which lists some of the general benefits of an active lifestyle and healthy eating.

Now you that you better understand the why, you can be more successful with the how of behavior change.

LEARNING FROM YOUR PAST

Do you feel overwhelmed by the idea of making lifestyle changes? Many people do. But chances are you've already exchanged some bad habits for good ones. Maybe you stopped or cut back on smoking. Or perhaps you cut down your soda intake and started drinking more water. Don't just think in terms of health habits. Try to remember any positive behavior change. Maybe you learned to hang up your car keys in the same place so that you didn't have to waste time searching for them every morning. Remembering changes you've made in the past can help you build confidence in your ability to change your activity and eating habits now. You can learn from past changes—both your successes and your failures. You can then apply this knowledge to improving your health habits now.

Make a list of habits you have changed for the better—your own personal success stories. Try to remember how you changed. What helped you succeed and what got in your way? Did a family member or friend help you in some way? Did you write down goals or find creative ways to remind yourself to follow through? Think about two or three habits you've changed and fill in figure 1.2.

FIGURE 1.2
My Personal Success Story

Habits I've Changed

Sample: I stopped biting my fingernails.

1._____

2._____

3._____

Things That Helped Me Succeed

Sample: I rewarded myself with a professional manicure every time I went two weeks without biting my nails.

1._____

2._____

3._____

Things That Got in My Way

Sample: I didn't give myself another way to deal with nervous energy. Usually when I feel stressed, I bite my nails. Not having an alternative made it harder to stop.

1._____

2._____

3._____

Adapted, by permission, from S.N. Blair, et al., 2001, *Active living every day* (Champaign, IL: Human Kinetics), 3-4.

HOW MUCH IS ENOUGH?

You may have ideas about what constitutes healthy eating and healthy activity levels. Magazines, newspapers, and television give us messages about the latest diets or the newest research on nutrition. You may have also picked up ideas from the people around you—family, friends, teachers, or coaches. Some of this information may be helpful, some misguided. Separating fact from fiction is important when trying to attain a healthy lifestyle.

To become aware of your beliefs about living a healthy lifestyle, take a moment to answer the 10 questions in figure 1.3. (You can check your answers on page 14.)

FIGURE 1.3
Lifestyle Quiz

Circle the letter (T for true and F for false) that you think most accurately represents each of the following 10 statements.

T   F   1. Physical activity has to be difficult to produce any benefits.

T   F   2. The only physical activities that count are structured exercises like jogging or strength training.

T   F   3. I can get health benefits from physical activity even if I do only a little, say 10 minutes, at a time.

T   F   4. Physical activities I do at home or work, like raking the leaves or taking the stairs instead of the elevator, count.

T   F   5. As long as I fit in a lot of physical activity over the weekend, I don't have to do anything else the rest of the week.

T   F   6. It's OK to eat any food I like, even rich foods like french fries or ice cream, as long as I do so in moderation.

T   F   7. The most successful diets restrict certain types of foods like carbohydrate.

T   F   8. It doesn't really matter what I eat, as long as I take the right supplements.

T   F   9. Drinking cranberry-apple juice is just as good for me as eating an apple.

T   F   10. Eating a variety of foods within each food group is important for good health.

Now that you've explored your own beliefs about healthy eating and physical activity, let's look at the current official guidelines for these health behaviors. Respected experts and agencies have established the following guidelines that are based on reliable research.

Physical Activity: The Real Deal

Did you check your answers to the Lifestyle Quiz? Were you surprised by any of the correct answers? Let's take a better look at what you actually need to do to stay healthy or improve your health. Although it may seem that everyone is confused about how much activity you need, experts in most developed countries agree on these principles:

> In the Surgeon General's Report on Physical Activity and Health (U.S. Department of Health and Human Services 1996), the U.S. surgeon general issued the following guidelines based on a review of more than 10 years of research on health and exercise: "All Americans should engage in regular physical activity at a level appropriate to their needs and interests. Significant health benefits can be obtained by setting and reaching a goal of accumulating at least 30 minutes of moderate-intensity physical activity on most, preferably all, days of the week. Those who currently meet these standards may derive additional benefits by becoming more physically active or including more vigorous activity."

Notice two key phrases in this statement: moderate-intensity physical activity and accumulate 30 minutes. Let's look at these more closely.

❋ An example of a moderate-intensity physical activity is a brisk walk, or walking 1 mile (1.6 kilometers) in 15 to 20 minutes (3 to 4 miles, or 4.8 to 6.4 kilometers, in an hour). That's a pace at which you'll likely feel invigorated. Your heart rate increases and you breathe more rapidly, but you can still carry on a conversation. Imagine you're walking to catch a bus you're a little late for. Many activities are moderately intense, such as dancing, raking leaves, low-impact aerobics, brisk treadmill walking, and golfing without a cart. For more examples of moderate-intensity activities, see appendix A.

❋ Research has shown that accumulating 30 minutes of moderate-intensity activity improves health. In other words, you don't have to do that activity all at once. Three 10-minute bouts of moderately intense exercise can reap health benefits similar to those from one 30-minute session. That's encouraging news for busy people who have a hard time fitting physical activity into their daily lives. You may not have time for a 30-minute walk, but you could probably fit in 10 minutes before work, 10 minutes at lunchtime, and 10 minutes after dinner.

What About Vigorous Activity?

You may be wondering about the role of vigorous activity. If you are already moderately active, doing more vigorous forms of activity, such as running, shoveling snow, circuit strength training, step aerobics, or playing tennis, can be a way to further improve your health and to add more interest and challenge to your routine. Research shows, however, that moderate activity is the best place to start for most inactive people. See appendix B for guidelines and a list of vigorous activities.

Healthy Eating: All Foods Can Fit

Are you confused about how to eat for good health? If you are, you are not alone. There's a myriad of information available in the media—some true, some false, and some downright dangerous. Knowing how to sort through all this information is important.

As with physical activity, the health agencies in most developed countries agree on what constitutes balanced eating. The developers of our Healthy Eating Every Day program have created an easy-to-use pyramid that reflects the latest reliable guidelines as endorsed by the USDA Dietary Guidelines for Americans and the public health guiding principles established in many developed countries. (See figure 1.4.)

Let's talk about the pyramid from the bottom up. Each recommendation is based on your daily needs.

Physical Activity

30 minutes

Notice that physical activity, at least 30 minutes a day, is an important part of healthy eating every day. Being physically active helps you maintain energy balance

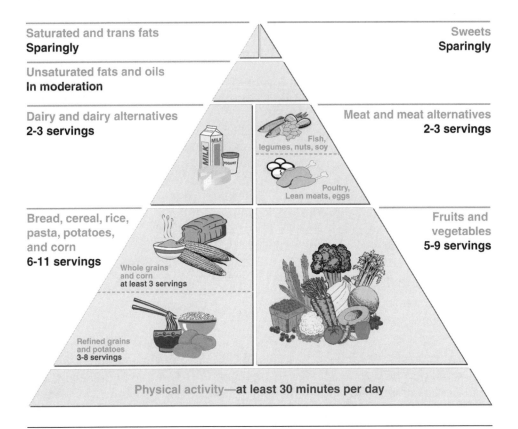

Figure 1.4 Healthy Eating Every Day pyramid of guidelines.

Reprinted, by permission, from R. Carpenter and C. Finley, 2005, *Healthy eating every day* (Champaign, IL: Human Kinetics), 5.

between the calories burned each day and those taken in through food. Good energy balance is key to maintaining a healthy weight.

Bread, Cereal, Rice, Pasta, Potato, and Corn Group (Grains)

6 to 11 servings

The largest food group is the one that contains breads, grains, pasta, potatoes, and corn. (Corn and potatoes are vegetables, but they are in the grain group because their nutritional makeup is more like that of the grain group.)

Within this group, there's a distinction between whole-grain foods and refined-grain foods and potatoes. Whole-grain foods (e.g., whole-grain breads and brown rice) have more fiber, vitamins, minerals, and phytochemicals (pronounced fight-o-chemicals). Phytochemicals are thought to help fight cancer and heart disease. Refined-grain foods (e.g., white bread and white rice) don't have much fiber or as much nutritional value as whole-grain foods. But all grain group foods are part of the foundation of a healthy diet.

Fruit and Vegetable Group

5 to 9 servings

Fruits and vegetables have lots of similar nutrients, so they are grouped together. They are rich sources of nutrients and fiber. On any given day, you can be flexible in how your fruit and vegetable servings stack up. For instance, one day you might eat one piece of fruit for breakfast and have five or six servings of vegetables during lunch and dinner. Another day you may have more fruit and fewer vegetables. Most adults do not get the recommended amounts of fruits and vegetables, so they're missing out on lots of good nutrition.

Meat and Meat Alternative Group

2 to 3 servings

Meat and meat alternatives are good sources of protein, and many of them contain iron and zinc. The Healthy Eating Every Day pyramid divides this group into two subcategories: those foods that have more saturated fat and cholesterol and those that have less saturated fat and cholesterol. Saturated fat and cholesterol can increase the level of cholesterol in your blood and may increase your risk for heart disease. Fish, legumes, nuts, and soy foods tend to be low in saturated fat and cholesterol. Beef, pork, lamb, chicken, and eggs are higher in saturated fat and cholesterol. If you are a vegetarian or don't eat certain forms of meat, please note that several meat alternatives are listed.

Dairy and Dairy Alternative Group

2 to 3 servings

Dairy products like milk, yogurt, and cheese and fortified dairy alternatives, such as soy milk, are the foods with the most calcium. Calcium is important for bone health and may help you maintain healthy blood pressure and body weight. The healthiest dairy and dairy alternatives are those that are low in fat. If you can't drink milk products, you can choose from several dairy alternatives. Be sure they are fortified with calcium.

Unsaturated Fat and Oil, Saturated and Trans Fat, and Sweets Groups

Use sparingly

The foods in these categories should be eaten in smaller amounts, even though some of them (unsaturated fat and oils) provide important nutrients. There are different types of fat and oils. Healthy oils include most vegetable oils, but especially canola, olive, and flaxseed oils. Soy, nuts, and fatty fish like salmon, mackerel, and herring also contain healthy oils.

Foods high in saturated and trans fat include butter, lard, whole milks and cheeses, most store-bought cookies, cakes, crackers, and chips, fried foods, and fatty cuts of meat. Since these foods may raise blood cholesterol, it's best to select lean varieties most often.

Sweet foods often have lots of calories and few nutrients. They are sometimes high in fat, too. Often called "empty-calorie" foods, chocolate, soda, cake, cookies, pie, sugar, honey, and jam should all be eaten sparingly.

For more information on serving sizes, see appendix D.

Balance, Variety, and Moderation

Besides knowing the specific types and amounts of foods you should eat, you should grasp three key principles of healthy eating: balance, variety, and moderation. These principles will help you to follow a diet that is healthy and enjoyable and suits your individual needs.

* Eating foods from all the food groups will ensure that you get the nutritional requirements for a strong body and good health. No single food group will give you all the nutrients your body needs. Nor is it healthy to completely eliminate an entire food group. For instance, low-carbohydrate, high-protein diets have been very popular in the past few years. But foods with carbohydrate such as whole grains provide important nutrients and fiber not found in high-protein foods.

* Within each food group, you need to eat a variety of foods. In other words, you may like apples and broccoli, but if you eat only those foods for your fruit and vegetable requirement, you will be missing many other valuable nutrients. It's important to expand your choices. For instance, oranges and grapefruit have much more vitamin C than apples. And carrots have lots of vitamin A and carotene. You don't have to know about all the vitamins, minerals, and phytochemicals in foods; simply look for variety in colors and shapes to ensure that you're getting a balance of nutrients. For more information visit www.5aday.gov.

* If you follow the principles of balance and variety, you will be eating lots of healthy foods. You may wonder whether there's a place for less healthy items such as rich desserts or fried foods. Yes, as long as you eat them in moderation. No single food is going to kill you or ensure perfect health. But the more whole (unprocessed), healthy foods you eat, the more likely you are to enjoy good health.

Let's look at an example. An apple is a whole food. Apple pie takes apples and combines them with lots of sugar and fat, so it's not considered a whole food, and it's not as healthy for you as an apple. But that doesn't mean that you should never eat apple pie. To maintain a healthy diet, it's better to eat a lot more apples and eat apple pie only for special occasions.

HOW CAN YOU IMPROVE?

Now that you've reviewed the guidelines on physical activity and healthy eating, what's your reaction? Did you learn anything new? Were you surprised by any of the guidelines? How do you see yourself and your habits in relation to these guidelines? Look at the guidelines and think about the foods you eat. Do you eat something from every category? Do you tend to eat mostly from two or three categories? Which ones dominate your food choices?

What about the amount and type of physical activity you get every day? Are you a very sedentary person? (Do you sit, drive, or stand most of the day?) Or are you somewhat active, perhaps getting some exercise on the weekends by doing chores or playing a sport? Starting to think about these things, even if you haven't made many improvements in your behavior yet, will help you as you go through the next three steps to healthy living.

Using Your First Steps Journal

To become more aware of where you stand right now and what steps you might want to take in the future, you can start using the First Steps Journal in part II of this book. Instead of trying to make changes right away, you should first determine exactly what you are eating every day and how active you are by recording everything in your journal. The journal is an excellent way to build your awareness about your healthy (or not-so-healthy) habits.

1. Track your eating habits. The section of the journal entitled My Healthy Eating Journal allows you to keep track of all the areas of healthy eating outlined in this chapter as well as servings and calories.

2. Track your physical activity. The physical activity section of your First Steps Journal gives you a variety of ways to add up the amount of time you spend being physically active in a day.

You can record vigorous activities and moderate activities that you engage in. You can also record lifestyle activities, like walking to work or washing windows. And you can record more structured activities, like swimming laps or running on a treadmill.

In addition, you'll find that you can set weekly goals, list the barriers to healthy habits that you want to address, and create motivational affirmations for yourself. You'll find more information about using your First Steps Journal in the section titled How to Use This Journal on page 37.

Most people have a good idea of how they should eat and know that they should be physically active. The problem is the daily hassles and obstacles that create barriers to healthy living.

Here are some common things people say when asked why they aren't more physically active or why they don't eat well:

"I don't have time."

"I hate to sweat."

"I don't get the support I need."

"I don't have much self-discipline."

In figure 1.5 list what you think may be some of the biggest barriers you'll meet when you try to be more active during your day or eat more healthfully. Be as specific as you can. For instance, "I don't have anyone to watch the baby while I go for a walk" might be one of your obstacles to activity. "My husband hates vegetables" may be a real obstacle when you prepare dinner. Don't judge or analyze your reasons. Be honest. What stops you? Once you know some of your barriers, you can start building solutions to overcome them.

FIGURE 1.5

My Barriers to Physical Activity and Healthy Eating

Barriers to Physical Activity

1._____

2._____

3._____

4._____

5._____

Barriers to Healthy Eating

1._____

2._____

3._____

4._____

5._____

Congratulations. In step 1 you have increased your awareness of what you hope to gain from a healthier lifestyle, learned from your past successes and disappointments, and explored your barriers to healthy habits. By doing this, you have built a strong foundation for step 2, creating solutions to your barriers to a healthy lifestyle.

Answers to Lifestyle Quiz

1. False. Research shows that regular moderate activity such as brisk walking can give you significant health benefits. And moderate activity is a better place for most inactive people to start (Blair, et. al. 1989).

2. False. Both structured activities such as jogging and lifestyle activity such as mowing the lawn can be counted in your daily accumulation of 30 minutes of activity. That's good news for busy people.

3. True. Studies have shown that accumulating activity in 10-minute bouts throughout the day results in similar health benefits as 30 minutes of nonstop activity (Debusk, et. al. 1990).

4. True. As mentioned in the answer to question 2, lifestyle activities of moderate intensity can improve health.

5. False. The public health guidelines indicate that to reap significant benefits you should accumulate 30 minutes of moderate-intensity activity at least 5 days a week. People who do vigorous activity (such as running) can do their activity 3 to 5 days a week.

6. True. Nutrition experts such as the researchers at the American Dietetic Association strongly promote the idea that all foods fit. As long as you are getting all the nutrients you need by eating a variety of foods from all the food groups, and don't overeat sweets, fat, and other less healthful foods, you should be fine.

7. False. One of the guiding principles of good nutrition is balance. It's important to eat foods from all the food groups so that you get all the nutrients you need for good health.

8. False. Some supplements such as a daily multivitamin can be helpful, but supplements should not replace real food in your diet.

9. False. Dietary guidelines encourage people to eat whole foods rather than depend on supplements. Although cranberry-apple juice may have the same vitamin content as an apple, the apple also has fiber. In addition, the juice is higher in sugar, so the apple is the healthier choice.

10. True. Even within the same food group, such as the fruit and vegetable group, different foods provide different nutrients, so you need to eat a variety of foods within each food group.

References

Blair, S.N., et. al. 1989. "Physical fitness and all-cause mortality: A prospective study of healthy men and women." *Journal of the American Medical Association* 262: 2395-2401.

Debusk, R.F., et. al. 1990. "Training effects of long versus short bouts of exercise in healthy subjects." *American Journal of Cardiology* 65 (15):1010-1013.

U.S. Department of Health and Human Services. 1996. *Physical activity and health: A report of the surgeon general.* Atlanta: U.S. Department of Health and Human Services, Centers for Disease Control and Prevention, National Center for Chronic Disease Prevention and Health Promotion. Available at www.cdc.gov/nccdphp/sgr/sgr.htm.

Step Two

CREATE
SOLUTIONS

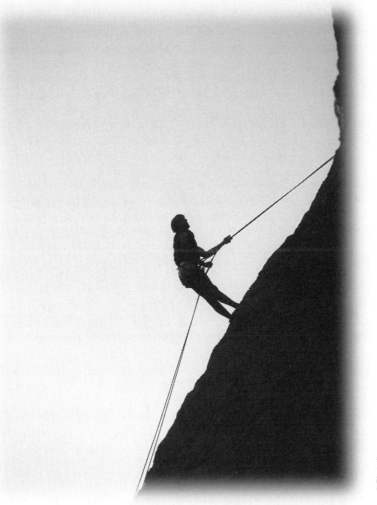

© Photodisc

"*M*ake it a practice to keep on the lookout for novel and interesting ideas that others have used successfully. Your idea only has to be original in its adaptation to the problem you are working on."

—*Thomas Edison*

Now that you've increased your awareness of your current health practices, let's move on to step 2, creating solutions to the things that are keeping you from attaining the healthy lifestyle you want. One of the best ways to predict whether you will be able to adopt and maintain a new health habit is to look at your perceived barriers and benefits to that habit. The fewer barriers you have, and the more benefits you can think of, the more likely you are to maintain your new health habit. So, learning to overcome barriers through problem solving is a way to reduce the barriers to behavior change. In step 2 you'll build specific skills related to overcoming barriers by learning to do the following:

* Understand the role of problem solving and why learning this skill is an important way to permanently overcome your barriers to healthy habits.
* Learn a simple problem-solving technique called the IDEA strategy.

IMPORTANCE OF PROBLEM SOLVING

Rather than give you a list of various solutions for common barriers (such as getting up earlier or giving up your least favorite TV show to solve the barrier of lack of time), this chapter teaches you some problem-solving skills to empower you in two important ways:

1. By problem-solving your own barriers, you will customize your solutions to your individual personality and lifestyle. No one solution is right for everyone. Think of it this way: If you come to a brick wall, there are many ways to get past it—dig under it, climb over it with a ladder, knock a hole in it, throw a rope over the top with a grappling hook, and so on. You need to find the way that makes the most sense for you and the tools at your disposal.

2. Your barriers to healthy living will change over time, depending on things such as the time of year, what's going on in your life right now, and your general life stage. For example, barriers for college students are different than those for parents of young children. By learning how to find different and creative ways of approaching the barriers (problem solving), you'll have powerful tools to address obstacles now and in the future.

We'd like you to approach problem solving as an experiment in healthy living, a creative process that you test until you get the results you want. Finding the right solution may take some time, but if you follow this plan, you're bound to see progress.

THE GREAT IDEA

The tool that we use in our Active Living Every Day and Healthy Eating Every Day courses is called the Great IDEA. The Great IDEA is a simple four-stage process for creating solutions to your barriers to healthy living. The acronym IDEA stands for the following:

- ❋ I for *identify* a barrier you want to work on
- ❋ D for *develop* a list of possible solutions
- ❋ E for *evaluate* a consideration of your possible solutions and a choice of the one solution you will try
- ❋ A for *analyze* your chosen solution after you've tried it

Here's how it works:

I – Identify the Problem

First, you have to recognize a problem so that you know what to work on. You're ahead of the game because you've already listed some of your barriers in step 1. Choose one that you'd like to work on and write it in figure 2.1 (see page 20). Reflect carefully on how or why this barrier operates in your life. Write down notes about the specifics of your personal barrier that help you to understand that barrier in detail.

Sample Barrier

> I can't be physically active because the weather is cold and snowy. I don't like being cold, and I feel unsafe when I'm walking on roads that are slippery.

D – Develop a List of Solutions

Now, create a list of all the ways you can think of to overcome the barrier you chose. Set your mind free to roam a bit. Take a few deep breaths, put on some relaxing music, and brainstorm about various solutions to your problem. You can do this alone or with a friend. Don't analyze your solutions yet. Make a list of everything that comes to mind, no matter how silly it may seem. Sometimes the best solutions may seem strange at first. Or, an idea you come up with may not be the perfect solution, but it may inspire another, more practical idea.

Sample List of Solutions

> - Move to Hawaii.
> - Buy good winter clothing and boots to wear when walking outside.
> - Set up and tend to an indoor garden.
> - Walk at the mall.
> - Get an exercise video and do it at home.

E - Evaluate Your Solutions

At this point, you can start to look at your solutions more critically. Notice which ones seem realistic and appealing to you. Some that at first appeared funny might seem pretty useful. Choose just one that you're willing to try for a week. Develop a specific plan for carrying it out.

Sample Evaluation

- Moving to Hawaii is tempting, but I can't afford it. Also, my family is here.
- I don't like the idea of buying winter clothing and boots because I don't like putting on all those extra clothes.
- I like the idea of gardening, but it's not a moderate-intensity activity.
- I like mall walking, but I don't want to have to clean off my car or drive on icy roads.

**I like the video solution because not only do I not have to be cold and uncomfortable for my activity, but I also don't have to shovel my driveway or scrape off my car as I would if I walked at the mall. Also, I know of a video I think I will like—I saw it at my friend's house. I choose to buy a physical activity video and do it at home as my solution. I will purchase my video this weekend, and I will do the video at home next week on Monday, Wednesday, and Friday.

A - Analyze How Well Your Plan Worked

Try your plan for a week. Make adjustments if necessary as you learn more about your barrier. Then take a look at how well it worked. Be honest. Make revisions to your plan, or throw out that idea and try another. Remember, you're experimenting, not failing. Think of this as a game, and the only way to lose is to give up.

Sample Analysis

My plan worked OK, but not as well as I hoped. I bought the video. I did it once, but then I skipped the other two days. I think I'd be more likely to do the video if I had someone to do it with me. I will ask a friend in my building to join me next week.

FIGURE 2.1
Great IDEAs

I

Identify the barriers you want to work on.

_____

_____

_____

_____

D

Develop a list of solutions.

_____

_____

_____

_____

E

Evaluate your solutions and choose one you are willing to try.

_____

_____

_____

_____

A

Analyze how well your plan worked.

_____

_____

_____

_____

Once you are comfortable using the Great IDEA, you can apply it whenever difficult situations arise. Our Active Living Every Day and Healthy Eating Every Day participants tell us that using the Great IDEA builds their self-confidence in overcoming their barriers to healthy living. Many people have even reported that they use the technique in other areas of their lives. As you continue to problem-solve individual barriers, your total list of barriers will decrease, improving your chances of long-term success.

You've just learned one of the most important tools for permanently improving your health. Barriers to healthy living will always exist. But you can learn to overcome the barriers and to view those barriers differently. By learning problem-solving skills, you can empower yourself to confidently deal with whatever obstacles come your way. Now let's move on to step 3, where you will discover how to boost your self-confidence and motivate yourself to stick with your new healthy habits.

References

Blair, S.N., A.L. Dunn, B.H. Marcus, R.A. Carpenter, and P. Jaret. 2001. *Active living every day.* Champaign, IL: Human Kinetics.

Carpenter, R.A. and C.E. Finley. 2005. *Healthy eating every day.* Champaign, IL: Human Kinetics.

Adapted, by permission, from S.N. Blair, et al., 2001, *Active living every day* (Champaign, IL: Human Kinetics), 30-31.

Step Three

BOOST
CONFIDENCE

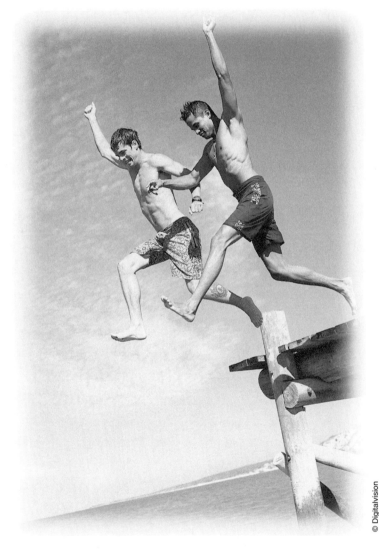

"Believe in yourself and you will be unstoppable."
—Emily Guay

Y ou can have the best plan in the world, but if you don't believe you can accomplish it, you won't get very far. In step 3, you will learn how to build confidence in your ability to make healthy changes. You will increase your sense of "I can do this!" You will discover how to silence that little voice in your head that says, "I can't do that" as you learn to replace "I can't" internal messages with more realistic, helpful thoughts.

Specifically, you will learn to do the following:

❋ Understand how your thoughts, emotions, and behaviors affect one another and identify and evaluate self-defeating thoughts that hinder your ability to stay on track.

❋ Learn to change your outlook.

UNDERSTANDING THOUGHT, EMOTION, AND BEHAVIOR

Here are some examples of how negative thinking can trip you up. You might set goals and build enthusiasm, and then you might inadvertently sabotage your success by letting habitual, self-defeating thoughts get the best of you. You might write positive goals, but a little voice in your head says, "I'll never be able to do this." You make a mistake or miss one daily goal, and you say, "See! I knew I couldn't do this."

Your thoughts, emotions, and behaviors constantly affect one another. These interactions come in different forms and can influence your health behaviors positively or negatively. Let's look at different ways this can happen:

Emotion → Thought → Behavior

1. After an argument with your teenage child you feel angry and upset (emotion).
2. You think, *I'm too upset to make breakfast* (thought).
3. You grab a doughnut instead of having a healthy breakfast (behavior).

Thought → Emotion → Behavior

1. You think, *I don't have time to make breakfast* (thought).
2. You feel guilty that you are not meeting your commitment (emotion).
3. You grab a doughnut to soothe yourself (behavior).

Behavior → Emotion → Thought

1. You flop on the couch or grab a doughnut (behavior).
2. You feel guilty (emotion).
3. You think, *I just can't change!* (thought).

We often feel helpless as we try to change our health habits, and we get caught in negative thinking patterns. You don't have to be trapped in this process, however. By learning to observe your thoughts and actions and change negative, unrealistic, or unhelpful thoughts as they arise, you can create a more positive outcome. Let's look at our first example again.

> After an argument with your teenage child, you feel angry and upset (emotion). You think, *I'm too upset to make breakfast* (unrealistic, unhelpful thought) and then catch yourself and reframe the thought: *That's not true. I am upset, but I can still pour myself a bowl of cereal and sit down to eat. Taking the time to eat breakfast will help me calm down. And I'll feel better about myself if I eat something healthy* (more realistic, helpful thought). You eat a bowl of cereal with fruit (positive behavior). As a result, you feel better about yourself (positive emotion).

So you see, the cycle of thoughts, emotions, and behaviors can have a positive or a negative result, depending on how you handle it. Changing the cycle takes time, but you can do it.

By learning to tune in to the false and unhelpful messages you send yourself, you can catch yourself in the act and turn that negative self-talk into more positive messages that can help you move forward. Here are some examples that illustrate how to reframe the different kinds of self-defeating thinking into more empowering thinking:

Exaggeration: "I just ate three candy bars. When it comes to healthy eating I'm a total failure."

Reframed thought: "OK. I ate the candy bars. But I'm not a total failure—that's an exaggeration. Actually, until I ate the candy bars, I ate quite well today. And over the last month, I've been consistently eating more fruits and vegetables as snacks. I can learn from this mistake and remember that sweets can be part of a healthy diet, as long as I eat them in smaller portions."

All-or-nothing thinking: "I skipped my walk again. I'll never be able to change."

Reframed thought: "*Never* is a pretty strong word. There are some obstacles to my being more physically active, but if I take things in small steps, I can slowly but consistently move toward reaching my goal. I'll schedule a walk for tomorrow and ask Sally to go with me."

Negative Thinking —It's Just a Bad Habit

Negative thoughts are most often the culprit that starts a downward cycle of feelings and behaviors. Most people engage in certain styles of thinking when they are trying to change their habits. Watch out for these unrealistic thought styles:

1. All-or-nothing thinking includes broad generalizations that use words such as *never* and *always*.

   Example: "I skipped my walk again. I'll never be able to change."

2. Exaggerating blows minor setbacks out of proportion.

   Example: "I just ate three candy bars. When it comes to healthy eating, I'm a total failure."

3. Faulty perceptions are false ideas about reality.

   Example: "I blew my whole plan for healthy eating at this picnic."

Faulty perceptions: "I blew my whole plan for healthy eating at this picnic."

Reframed thought: "That's not actually true. I did overeat. But I made some good choices (carrot sticks instead of potato salad), and I ate a very healthy breakfast today. This is just one meal on one day. I will do better tomorrow. And by using the IDEA strategy, I can plan how to overcome the temptation to overeat the next time I go to a family outing like this."

CHANGING YOUR OUTLOOK

You are the only person who can turn your self-defeating thoughts around, because you're the only one who hears them. It's up to you to be on the lookout for these kinds of thoughts and find ways to turn them into thoughts that support your desire for healthier habits. Here are the three steps you can use:

1. Identify self-defeating thoughts. Ask yourself whether your thoughts are having a negative influence on your feelings and actions. Watch for patterns of unhelpful thinking.

2. Evaluate self-defeating thoughts. Ask yourself whether your thoughts are based on truth or on reality. For instance, the statement "I haven't had any dairy foods all week. Now I'll get osteoporosis for sure" isn't based on reality.

3. Modify self-defeating thoughts. Replace your self-defeating thoughts with more empowering (and realistic) ones. For example, "I haven't eaten my dairy servings this week, but I plan on stocking my refrigerator with lots of dairy options for next week."

Now, take a few minutes to think of a familiar message you tend to give yourself. Record your message in figure 3.1.

Learning to reframe your thoughts so that they work *for* you, not against you, takes time and practice. Your brain has gotten into some unhelpful thinking patterns, and it will take awhile to get in the habit of thinking more realistically. But

---

FIGURE 3.1

Message to Myself

Identify the self-defeating thought:

_____

Evaluate that message and ask yourself if it's based on reality:

_____

Modify the message so that it is more realistic and empowering:

_____

---

it is possible, so keep at it. You can actually have fun catching yourself in the act of self-defeating thinking and turning those negative thoughts into positive and empowering messages.

You're doing great! Now you know how to silence your biggest critic—you—and train your mind to send positive thoughts that will set you up for success. That, along with building awareness and being able to problem-solve your barriers to healthy living, will take you a long way toward creating the healthy lifestyle you desire. Now that you've taken the steps to build awareness, create solutions, and boost confidence, let's take a look at how you can sustain your commitment to your new behaviors over time.

Step Four

SUSTAIN COMMITMENT

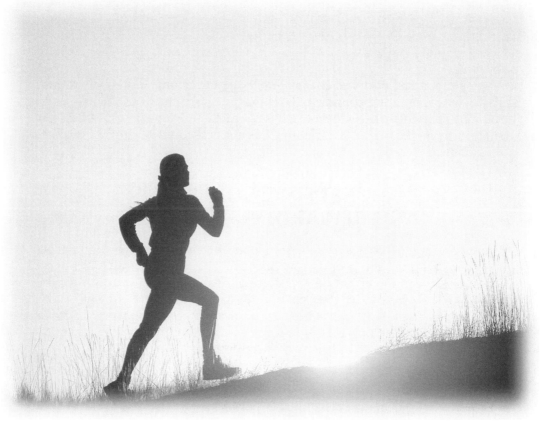

"You've got to think about the 'big things' while you are doing the small things so that all the small things go in the right direction."

—*Alvin Toffler*

Every January millions of people around the world make resolutions to change some aspect of their behaviors. Amidst the New Year's celebrations, or perhaps during a quiet moment alone, they dedicate themselves to a worthy goal with positive intention and great hope. And by February, they've run out of steam. "I tried," they may say, "but it didn't work out."

Step 4 is about making your lifestyle changes permanent. The behavior changes you want to make are not for a week or a month or even a year. They're commitments to a healthier way of living for the rest of your life. While your enthusiasm may be high right now, we know you'll need strategies to keep going after the initial motivation wears off.

In step 4, you'll learn to sustain commitment by discovering how to

* set effective goals, distinguish between short-term goals and long-term goals, and reward yourself along the way, and
* monitor your progress.

People honestly do try to change, but when they stumble, they often quit. That's where building commitment comes in. It's difficult to change long-standing habits. Patience with yourself is essential. And knowing that when you slip you are not failing but participating in a normal process of growth can mean the difference between success and failure.

SETTING GOALS
AND REWARDING YOURSELF

People who set goals are more successful at making lasting changes than people who don't set goals. But people don't often talk about their personal or professional goals. You might not be accustomed to talking about goals, or maybe you don't know how to set good goals. And chances are you're not good about rewarding yourself. Let's look at the goal-setting process and the importance of rewards. Then we'll talk about self-monitoring, the skill that helps you stay on track to meet those goals and enjoy those rewards.

Goals

An effective goal has four core characteristics:

1. Personal
2. Realistic
3. Specific
4. Measurable

If any of these core characteristics is missing, your goal may be too difficult to reach or to track, and your success may be hindered. Let's look at each element separately.

1. **Personal.** By this, we mean that the goal meets your needs and desires. Unfortunately, sometimes you might set goals to please others; rarely are those goals realized. To be successful, you have to set your own goal, and the goal has to be something you truly want to achieve.

* **Impersonal goal:** My husband wants me to exercise more.

* **Personal goal:** I know that physical activity is good for my body, my health, and my sense of well-being. I would love to be more active and reap those rewards. I plan to add 10 minutes to my usual walking routine and pick up the pace so that I'm walking more briskly.

2. **Realistic.** Your goal needs to be challenging but attainable. If it's too difficult, you'll fail; if it's too easy, you won't pay attention to it. You may need to learn more about your goal to determine if it's actually attainable for you. You can determine this by asking your doctor, a teacher, or a knowledgeable friend or family member.

* **Unrealistic goal:** Next week I will run 5 miles a day for health and fitness (if you are sedentary and not used to running).

* **Realistic goal:** I know that the benefits of vigorous exercise are more energy and endurance and better health. But I need to work up to running. This week I will start by walking 10 minutes a day at least three days during the week.

3. **Specific.** You may have noticed in the previous examples that the goal was clearly stated in specific terms. Vague statements about what you want to accomplish lead to vague plans or no plans at all.

* **Vague goal:** I will eat more healthfully.

* **Specific goal:** I will eat fresh fruit with breakfast daily.

4. **Measurable.** Once you have a personal, realistic, specific goal, you need to decide how you will measure your success. This is where your First Steps Journal really helps you. Let's look at the previous example:

* **Immeasurable goal:** I will eat more fruit at breakfast.

* **Measurable goal:** I will eat fresh fruit at breakfast every day. I will measure this by noting my servings in my First Steps Journal.

As you think about the goals you want to set, classify them as short-term goals or long-term goals. A long-term goal reflects what you ultimately want to achieve. Short-term goals, though perhaps less glamorous, are the steps that get you there. Long-term goals may take a month or many months to accomplish. Short-term goals are accomplished on a weekly basis, day by day. Here's a sample of related long-term and short-term goals:

* **Long-term goal:** I will eat 5 servings of fruit and vegetables every day, which will be confirmed in my First Steps Journal.

* **Short-term goal:** This week, I will buy enough fruit on Sunday to have a serving with breakfast every day. I will record eating fruit for breakfast in my First Steps Journal.

Rewards

Studies show that rewarding yourself for positive behaviors can help you build commitment to the goal and reach the goal. You might be happy to reward your friends, spouses, or other loved ones when you reach a goal or achieve something in your life, but maybe you don't think of rewarding yourself for the same accomplishments. Rewards help you to stay focused and maintain enthusiasm for your goals when you encounter difficult times. You don't have to save your reward for the long-term goal. You can reward yourself every step of the way.

Be creative in choosing your rewards. They can be material things, like buying a new CD or going to a movie. Or your rewards can be intangible (meaning you can't touch it physically), such as giving yourself permission to sleep late on Saturday or talking on the phone with an old friend you've lost touch with.

Make sure you choose rewards that move your goals forward rather than backward. For instance, don't promise yourself an ice cream sundae for eating healthier breakfasts. You might consider rewarding yourself with a juicer or some fresh oranges direct from Florida. If you're working on your physical activity goals, a great reward might be a massage or a bubble bath or a new, easy-care haircut.

Now that you understand the value of long-term and short-term goals and the value of rewarding yourself for positive behavior changes, take a moment to reflect on the process and come up with one long-term goal and one short-term goal and write them down.

Test the goals against the four criteria for effective goals: Are the goals personal, realistic, specific, and measurable? Decide how you will reward yourself when you achieve the goals. Make sure your short-term goal is something that moves your long-term goal forward. Record your goals in figure 4.1.

Use your First Steps Journal to record your goals, whether for a week, several weeks, or a month or more. Include a note to yourself so that when you've reached a specific goal, you know it's time to follow up with that well-earned reward.

MONITORING YOUR HABITS: THE KEY TO SUCCESS

We devoted more than half of this book to space for a journal because studies show that people who regularly track their eating and physical activity make better progress in reaching their health goals. Occasionally things will happen that will shake your life up, and goals may fall by the wayside. If you're only looking at what's happening in the moment, you may become discouraged. By using the journal in the back of this book, you'll have a record that you can look to when things are going well—and when they aren't. You can keep the bigger picture in front of you and see all your accomplishments in black and white. (It's so easy to forget the great changes you've made when you're upset about what you haven't accomplished.) You can also use this information to fine-tune your plans.

By taking the time to study the four steps to successful behavior change for health, you are well on the way to reaching your healthy living goals. Now, be sure to move to part II of this book, where you'll find further instructions for

FIGURE 4.1
Goals

*Long-Term Goal*_____

Personal? Yes, because_____.

Realistic? Yes, because_____.

Specific? Yes, because_____.

Measurable? Yes. I will measure it by_____.

I will reward myself by_____.

*Short-Term Goal*_____

Will this help me attain my long-term goal? How?_____

_____.

Personal? Yes, because_____.

Realistic? Yes, because_____.

Specific? Yes, because_____.

Measurable? Yes. I will measure it by_____.

I will reward myself by_____.

using your First Steps Journal to monitor your progress effectively. And remember that healthy living is a journey; people move back and forth between success and temporary setbacks. Refer to the four steps often so that you keep using these important lifestyle skills and stay on track. Good luck!

MOVING FORWARD

We hope you have enjoyed learning the four steps to changing your health habits, and we hope that you will continue to make progress by using the journal section of this book. If you would like to learn more and have even more support to reach your goals, you may want to consider two exceptional tools available to you. Active Living Partners has produced two complete and detailed courses, Active Living Every Day and Healthy Eating Every Day. These courses were developed and tested at The Cooper Institute and are full of proven strategies and tips for improving your health and well-being.

Active Living Every Day

Active Living Every Day will help you become and stay physically active. Besides gaining more details on the tools we've presented in *First Steps*, you will learn about additional tools to help you be more active:

* Manage time to fit activity into your busy schedule.
* Overcome lapses in activity.
* Discover activities you enjoy and will stick with.
* Deal with people who try to undermine your attempt to be physically active.

Healthy Eating Every Day

Address the real causes of your unhealthy eating habits and find the tools you need to succeed in eating better with Healthy Eating Every Day. In addition to learning more about the four steps presented in *First Steps*, you will discover how to do the following:

* Choose the right balance of the right foods for optimal health.
* Cope with triggers to unhealthy eating.
* Eat well at home, at work, and when traveling or dining out.
* Make healthy food choices even when you are in a hurry.

Learning activities, stories about real-life people, and resource guides will help you every step of the way. These programs were tested with real people just like you to create state-of-the-art, practical guidance. You can take Active Living Partners courses with a licensed provider in your community or online on your own. For more information, visit www.ActiveLiving.info or call 800-747-4457.

Part Two

❧

FIRST STEPS
JOURNAL

HOW TO USE THIS JOURNAL

Y our First Steps Journal is designed to fit your needs, whether you are just beginning your journey to a healthier lifestyle or if you are looking to reach a higher level of health and fitness. The following explains how to use your First Steps Journal in a way that will work best for you.

Your First Steps Journal has weekly two-page spreads for you to use. Each two-page spread is divided into three distinct sections: healthy eating, physical activity, and behavior change skills. In addition we've provided a reproducible daily tracking form so you can easily monitor your eating and activity even when you're on the run.

HEALTHY EATING

You can track the following in the healthy eating section of your journal:

Servings by Food Group

It's easy to keep track of how many servings you eat within the following food groups:

* Fruits and vegetables
* Grains
* Dairy and dairy alternatives
* Meat and meat alternatives
* Fats
* Sweets

Simply write the total number of servings for each group in the boxes provided. To review recommended servings for all the food groups and how much of each food group is a serving, refer to appendix D, page 152.

Calories

If you are monitoring your weight, you may also want to track calories. To do this, track the calories for each serving of food you eat on your daily tracking form. At the end of the day, total up your calories and enter that amount in the total calories section.

A detailed discussion of weight management and calorie counting is beyond the scope of this book, but we have listed a number of good resources on page 159.

PHYSICAL ACTIVITY

You have several options on how to track your physical activity: minutes of exercise, activity, and steps per day.

Minutes of Moderate or Vigorous Intensity

Your First Steps Journal has places for you to enter both moderate-intensity and vigorous-intensity physical activity. Each time you are active, decide whether the activity is moderate or vigorous, and enter the number of minutes in that box.

For guidelines on moderate-intensity physical activity, refer to appendix A on page 147. For guidelines on vigorous-intensity activities, see appendix B on page 148. For examples of light, moderate, and vigorous activities, see appendix C on page 150.

Lifestyle or Structured Activities

Within both moderate and vigorous categories you can track lifestyle and structured activities. Lifestyle activities are activities that fit into your daily routine, like raking the leaves, playing outside with your kids, or taking the stairs instead of the elevator. Structured activities usually take a little more planning and include things like jogging, playing tennis, taking a Pilates class, or doing strength training. Both types of activity are health enhancing. The list of moderate and vigorous activities in appendix C (page 150) includes both lifestyle and structured activities.

Steps Per Day

Some people prefer to track steps per day rather than minutes. Step counters (small plastic devices attached to a belt worn over the hipbone) have become very popular. McDonald's even included step counters in their adult Happy Meals recently. You'll find a place to record your daily steps in the physical activity section of your First Steps Journal. For guidelines on steps per day, see appendix F on page 155.

BEHAVIOR CHANGE

One of the things that sets *First Steps* apart from other programs is that we not only give you reliable guidelines for physical activity and eating, but we also empower you to make those changes by providing practical tools to make behavior changes. You can track your use of the tools you learned in the first part of this book.

Setting Goals

In this section, you can enter a long- or short-term goal along with a reward you will give yourself when you meet that goal. To review effective goal setting and rewarding yourself, refer to step 4, starting on page 28.

Overcoming Barriers

Here you can write down a barrier you want to work on (from your list in step 1 or a new one you've encountered). Then enter your chosen strategy for overcoming that barrier. Don't forget to use the Great IDEA in step 2, starting on page 16.

Affirmations

You can fill out this section in a few ways:

1. Referring back to step 3 (starting on page 21) you can enter a self-defeating thought you wish to change and the empowering thought you plan to replace it with.
2. You can enter a personal mantra that will motivate you. Here are a couple examples: "Day by day I am honoring my body by making healthier food choices" and "I am increasing my energy by walking every day."
3. You can write down a quote that you find inspiring.

This is your space to use as you wish. Enter any other thoughts, helpful hints, or words of encouragement that will help you achieve a healthier lifestyle.

Daily Tracking Form

Some days you may want to keep track of your eating and physical activity in more detail or you may wish to use a smaller tracking tool that is easy to carry with you. The daily tracking form on page 41 is perfect for these situations (see sample on page 40). To use the form, simply photocopy the entire page and fold it in half. Your daily tracking form easily fits in your purse, pack, or briefcase, allowing you to make entries all day long.

Enter the information just as you would in the weekly tracking journal by listing the specific foods you ate or activities performed and their corresponding servings/calories or minutes/steps. At the end of the week transfer your totals onto the weekly tracking sheet so you can chart your overall weekly health habits.

HEALTHY EATING DAILY JOURNAL Date Monday	Calories	Servings					
		Fruits & Veggies	Grains	Dairy	Meats	Fats	Sweets
Breakfast: 1 cup Cheerios	111		2				
1/2 cup blueberries	41	1					
1 cup (1%) milk	102			1			
1/2 cup orange juice	55	1					
Lunch: Large fast-food burger with toppings	800		2		2	4	
Coffee w/ cream	40					1	
Dinner: 1 cup spaghetti	197		2				
1/2 cup sauce	80	1					
3 tbsp. parmesan cheese	66			1/2			
Salad with dressing	250	1				2	
Diet soda	0						
Snacks: 1 Snack-pack pudding	102			1			1
1 Candy bar	220						1
TOTAL	2064	4	6	2 1/2	2	7	2

PHYSICAL ACTIVITY DAILY JOURNAL Date Monday	Minutes	Number of steps	Calories burned
Morning: Parked couple blocks away from office	5	500	19
Afternoon: Brisk walk after lunch	10	1000	37
Evening: Walk back to car	5	500	19
Express strength-training circuit at club	25	?	226
* Includes total daily pedometer count **TOTAL**	45	8264*	301

HEALTHY EATING DAILY JOURNAL Date_____	Calories	Servings					
		Fruits & Veggies	Grains	Dairy	Meats	Fats	Sweets
Breakfast:							
Lunch:							
Dinner:							
Snacks:							
TOTAL							

PHYSICAL ACTIVITY DAILY JOURNAL Date_____	Minutes	Number of steps	Calories burned
Morning:			
Afternoon:			
Evening:			
TOTAL			

This is an original. Copy this form for your daily record keeping.

Week of _____

MY HEALTHY EATING JOURNAL

	Monday	Tuesday	Wednesday	Thursday	Friday	Saturday	Sunday
Servings eaten							
Fruits and vegetables							
Grains							
Dairy and dairy alternatives							
Meat and meat alternatives							
Fats							
Sweets							
Calories per day							

My plans

Goals:

Barriers/solutions:

Affirmations:

MY PHYSICAL ACTIVITY JOURNAL

	Monday	Tuesday	Wednesday	Thursday	Friday	Saturday	Sunday
Minutes of moderate exercise							
Lifestyle							
Structured							
Minutes of vigorous activity							
Lifestyle							
Structured							
Total minutes							
Total steps							

My plans

Goals:

Barriers/solutions:

Affirmations:

Week of _____

MY HEALTHY EATING JOURNAL

	Monday	Tuesday	Wednesday	Thursday	Friday	Saturday	Sunday
				Servings eaten			
Fruits and vegetables							
Grains							
Dairy and dairy alternatives							
Meat and meat alternatives							
Fats							
Sweets							
Calories per day							

My plans

Goals:

Barriers/solutions:

Affirmations:

MY PHYSICAL ACTIVITY JOURNAL

	Monday	Tuesday	Wednesday	Thursday	Friday	Saturday	Sunday
Minutes of moderate exercise							
Lifestyle							
Structured							
Minutes of vigorous activity							
Lifestyle							
Structured							
Total minutes							
Total steps							

My plans

Goals:

Barriers/solutions:

Affirmations:

Week of _____

MY HEALTHY EATING JOURNAL

	Monday	Tuesday	Wednesday	Thursday	Friday	Saturday	Sunday
				Servings eaten			
Fruits and vegetables							
Grains							
Dairy and dairy alternatives							
Meat and meat alternatives							
Fats							
Sweets							
Calories per day							

My plans

Goals:

Barriers/solutions:

Affirmations:

MY PHYSICAL ACTIVITY JOURNAL

	Monday	Tuesday	Wednesday	Thursday	Friday	Saturday	Sunday
Minutes of moderate exercise							
Lifestyle							
Structured							
Minutes of vigorous activity							
Lifestyle							
Structured							
Total minutes							
Total steps							

My plans
Goals:
Barriers/solutions:
Affirmations:

Week of _____

 MY HEALTHY EATING JOURNAL

	Monday	Tuesday	Wednesday	Thursday	Friday	Saturday	Sunday
				Servings eaten			
Fruits and vegetables							
Grains							
Dairy and dairy alternatives							
Meat and meat alternatives							
Fats							
Sweets							
Calories per day							

My plans

Goals:

Barriers/solutions:

Affirmations:

MY PHYSICAL ACTIVITY JOURNAL

	Monday	Tuesday	Wednesday	Thursday	Friday	Saturday	Sunday
Minutes of moderate exercise							
Lifestyle							
Structured							
Minutes of vigorous activity							
Lifestyle							
Structured							
Total minutes							
Total steps							

My plans

Goals:

Barriers/solutions:

Affirmations:

Week of _____

MY HEALTHY EATING JOURNAL

	Monday	Tuesday	Wednesday	Thursday	Friday	Saturday	Sunday
Servings eaten							
Fruits and vegetables							
Grains							
Dairy and dairy alternatives							
Meat and meat alternatives							
Fats							
Sweets							
Calories per day							

My plans

Goals:

Barriers/solutions:

Affirmations:

MY PHYSICAL ACTIVITY JOURNAL

	Monday	Tuesday	Wednesday	Thursday	Friday	Saturday	Sunday
Minutes of moderate exercise							
Lifestyle							
Structured							
Minutes of vigorous activity							
Lifestyle							
Structured							
Total minutes							
Total steps							

My plans

Goals:

Barriers/solutions:

Affirmations:

Week of _____

MY HEALTHY EATING JOURNAL

	Monday	Tuesday	Wednesday	Thursday	Friday	Saturday	Sunday
				Servings eaten			
Fruits and vegetables							
Grains							
Dairy and dairy alternatives							
Meat and meat alternatives							
Fats							
Sweets							
Calories per day							

My plans
Goals:
Barriers/solutions:
Affirmations:

MY PHYSICAL ACTIVITY JOURNAL

	Monday	Tuesday	Wednesday	Thursday	Friday	Saturday	Sunday
Minutes of moderate exercise							
Lifestyle							
Structured							
Minutes of vigorous activity							
Lifestyle							
Structured							
Total minutes							
Total steps							

My plans

Goals:

Barriers/solutions:

Affirmations:

Week of _____

MY HEALTHY EATING JOURNAL

	Monday	Tuesday	Wednesday	Thursday	Friday	Saturday	Sunday
				Servings eaten			
Fruits and vegetables							
Grains							
Dairy and dairy alternatives							
Meat and meat alternatives							
Fats							
Sweets							
Calories per day							

My plans

Goals:

Barriers/solutions:

Affirmations:

MY PHYSICAL ACTIVITY JOURNAL

	Monday	Tuesday	Wednesday	Thursday	Friday	Saturday	Sunday
Minutes of moderate exercise							
Lifestyle							
Structured							
Minutes of vigorous activity							
Lifestyle							
Structured							
Total minutes							
Total steps							

My plans

Goals:

Barriers/solutions:

Affirmations:

Week of _____

MY HEALTHY EATING JOURNAL

	Monday	Tuesday	Wednesday	Thursday	Friday	Saturday	Sunday
Servings eaten							
Fruits and vegetables							
Grains							
Dairy and dairy alternatives							
Meat and meat alternatives							
Fats							
Sweets							
Calories per day							

My plans

Goals:

Barriers/solutions:

Affirmations:

MY PHYSICAL ACTIVITY JOURNAL

	Monday	Tuesday	Wednesday	Thursday	Friday	Saturday	Sunday
Minutes of moderate exercise							
Lifestyle							
Structured							
Minutes of vigorous activity							
Lifestyle							
Structured							
Total minutes							
Total steps							

My plans

Goals:

Barriers/solutions:

Affirmations:

Week of _____

MY HEALTHY EATING JOURNAL

	Monday	Tuesday	Wednesday	Thursday	Friday	Saturday	Sunday
				Servings eaten			
Fruits and vegetables							
Grains							
Dairy and dairy alternatives							
Meat and meat alternatives							
Fats							
Sweets							
Calories per day							

My plans

Goals:

Barriers/solutions:

Affirmations:

MY PHYSICAL ACTIVITY JOURNAL

	Monday	Tuesday	Wednesday	Thursday	Friday	Saturday	Sunday
Minutes of moderate exercise							
Lifestyle							
Structured							
Minutes of vigorous activity							
Lifestyle							
Structured							
Total minutes							
Total steps							

My plans

Goals:

Barriers/solutions:

Affirmations:

Week of _____

MY HEALTHY EATING JOURNAL

	Monday	Tuesday	Wednesday	Thursday	Friday	Saturday	Sunday
				Servings eaten			
Fruits and vegetables							
Grains							
Dairy and dairy alternatives							
Meat and meat alternatives							
Fats							
Sweets							
Calories per day							

My plans

Goals:

Barriers/solutions:

Affirmations:

MY PHYSICAL ACTIVITY JOURNAL

	Monday	Tuesday	Wednesday	Thursday	Friday	Saturday	Sunday
Minutes of moderate exercise							
Lifestyle							
Structured							
Minutes of vigorous activity							
Lifestyle							
Structured							
Total minutes							
Total steps							

My plans

Goals:

Barriers/solutions:

Affirmations:

Week of _____

 # MY HEALTHY EATING JOURNAL

	Monday	Tuesday	Wednesday	Thursday	Friday	Saturday	Sunday
	Servings eaten						
Fruits and vegetables							
Grains							
Dairy and dairy alternatives							
Meat and meat alternatives							
Fats							
Sweets							
Calories per day							

My plans

Goals:

Barriers/solutions:

Affirmations:

MY PHYSICAL ACTIVITY JOURNAL

	Monday	Tuesday	Wednesday	Thursday	Friday	Saturday	Sunday
Minutes of moderate exercise							
Lifestyle							
Structured							
Minutes of vigorous activity							
Lifestyle							
Structured							
Total minutes							
Total steps							

My plans

Goals:

Barriers/solutions:

Affirmations:

Week of _____

MY HEALTHY EATING JOURNAL

	Monday	Tuesday	Wednesday	Thursday	Friday	Saturday	Sunday
				Servings eaten			
Fruits and vegetables							
Grains							
Dairy and dairy alternatives							
Meat and meat alternatives							
Fats							
Sweets							
Calories per day							

My plans

Goals:

Barriers/solutions:

Affirmations:

MY PHYSICAL ACTIVITY JOURNAL

	Monday	Tuesday	Wednesday	Thursday	Friday	Saturday	Sunday
Minutes of moderate exercise							
Lifestyle							
Structured							
Minutes of vigorous activity							
Lifestyle							
Structured							
Total minutes							
Total steps							

My plans

Goals:

Barriers/solutions:

Affirmations:

Week of _____

MY HEALTHY EATING JOURNAL

	Monday	Tuesday	Wednesday	Thursday	Friday	Saturday	Sunday
				Servings eaten			
Fruits and vegetables							
Grains							
Dairy and dairy alternatives							
Meat and meat alternatives							
Fats							
Sweets							
Calories per day							

My plans

Goals:

Barriers/solutions:

Affirmations:

MY PHYSICAL ACTIVITY JOURNAL

	Monday	Tuesday	Wednesday	Thursday	Friday	Saturday	Sunday
	Minutes of moderate exercise						
Lifestyle							
Structured							
	Minutes of vigorous activity						
Lifestyle							
Structured							
Total minutes							
Total steps							

My plans

Goals:

Barriers/solutions:

Affirmations:

Week of _____

	Monday	Tuesday	Wednesday	Thursday	Friday	Saturday	Sunday
				Servings eaten			
Fruits and vegetables							
Grains							
Dairy and dairy alternatives							
Meat and meat alternatives							
Fats							
Sweets							
Calories per day							

My plans

Goals:

Barriers/solutions:

Affirmations:

MY PHYSICAL ACTIVITY JOURNAL

	Monday	Tuesday	Wednesday	Thursday	Friday	Saturday	Sunday
Minutes of moderate exercise							
Lifestyle							
Structured							
Minutes of vigorous activity							
Lifestyle							
Structured							
Total minutes							
Total steps							

My plans

Goals:

Barriers/solutions:

Affirmations:

Week of _____

MY HEALTHY EATING JOURNAL

	Monday	Tuesday	Wednesday	Thursday	Friday	Saturday	Sunday
	Servings eaten						
Fruits and vegetables							
Grains							
Dairy and dairy alternatives							
Meat and meat alternatives							
Fats							
Sweets							
Calories per day							

My plans

Goals:

Barriers/solutions:

Affirmations:

MY PHYSICAL ACTIVITY JOURNAL

	Monday	Tuesday	Wednesday	Thursday	Friday	Saturday	Sunday
	Minutes of moderate exercise						
Lifestyle							
Structured							
	Minutes of vigorous activity						
Lifestyle							
Structured							
Total minutes							
Total steps							

My plans

Goals:

Barriers/solutions:

Affirmations:

Week of _____

MY HEALTHY EATING JOURNAL

	Monday	Tuesday	Wednesday	Thursday	Friday	Saturday	Sunday
				Servings eaten			
Fruits and vegetables							
Grains							
Dairy and dairy alternatives							
Meat and meat alternatives							
Fats							
Sweets							
Calories per day							

My plans

Goals:

Barriers/solutions:

Affirmations:

MY PHYSICAL ACTIVITY JOURNAL

	Monday	Tuesday	Wednesday	Thursday	Friday	Saturday	Sunday
Minutes of moderate exercise							
Lifestyle							
Structured							
Minutes of vigorous activity							
Lifestyle							
Structured							
Total minutes							
Total steps							

My plans

Goals:

Barriers/solutions:

Affirmations:

Week of _____

MY HEALTHY EATING JOURNAL

	Monday	Tuesday	Wednesday	Thursday	Friday	Saturday	Sunday
Servings eaten							
Fruits and vegetables							
Grains							
Dairy and dairy alternatives							
Meat and meat alternatives							
Fats							
Sweets							
Calories per day							

My plans

Goals:

Barriers/solutions:

Affirmations:

MY PHYSICAL ACTIVITY JOURNAL

	Monday	Tuesday	Wednesday	Thursday	Friday	Saturday	Sunday
Minutes of moderate exercise							
Lifestyle							
Structured							
Minutes of vigorous activity							
Lifestyle							
Structured							
Total minutes							
Total steps							

My plans

Goals:

Barriers/solutions:

Affirmations:

Week of _____

MY HEALTHY EATING JOURNAL

	Monday	Tuesday	Wednesday	Thursday	Friday	Saturday	Sunday
Servings eaten							
Fruits and vegetables							
Grains							
Dairy and dairy alternatives							
Meat and meat alternatives							
Fats							
Sweets							
Calories per day							

My plans
Goals:
Barriers/solutions:
Affirmations:

MY PHYSICAL ACTIVITY JOURNAL

	Monday	Tuesday	Wednesday	Thursday	Friday	Saturday	Sunday
	Minutes of moderate exercise						
Lifestyle							
Structured							
	Minutes of vigorous activity						
Lifestyle							
Structured							
Total minutes							
Total steps							

My plans

Goals:

Barriers/solutions:

Affirmations:

Week of _____

MY HEALTHY EATING JOURNAL

	Monday	Tuesday	Wednesday	Thursday	Friday	Saturday	Sunday
				Servings eaten			
Fruits and vegetables							
Grains							
Dairy and dairy alternatives							
Meat and meat alternatives							
Fats							
Sweets							
Calories per day							

My plans

Goals:

Barriers/solutions:

Affirmations:

MY PHYSICAL ACTIVITY JOURNAL

	Monday	Tuesday	Wednesday	Thursday	Friday	Saturday	Sunday
Minutes of moderate exercise							
Lifestyle							
Structured							
Minutes of vigorous activity							
Lifestyle							
Structured							
Total minutes							
Total steps							

My plans

Goals:

Barriers/solutions:

Affirmations:

Week of _____

MY HEALTHY EATING JOURNAL

	Monday	Tuesday	Wednesday	Thursday	Friday	Saturday	Sunday
	Servings eaten						
Fruits and vegetables							
Grains							
Dairy and dairy alternatives							
Meat and meat alternatives							
Fats							
Sweets							
Calories per day							

My plans
Goals:
Barriers/solutions:
Affirmations:

MY PHYSICAL ACTIVITY JOURNAL

	Monday	Tuesday	Wednesday	Thursday	Friday	Saturday	Sunday
Minutes of moderate exercise							
Lifestyle							
Structured							
Minutes of vigorous activity							
Lifestyle							
Structured							
Total minutes							
Total steps							

My plans

Goals:

Barriers/solutions:

Affirmations:

Week of _____

MY HEALTHY EATING JOURNAL

	Monday	Tuesday	Wednesday	Thursday	Friday	Saturday	Sunday
				Servings eaten			
Fruits and vegetables							
Grains							
Dairy and dairy alternatives							
Meat and meat alternatives							
Fats							
Sweets							
Calories per day							

My plans

Goals:

Barriers/solutions:

Affirmations:

MY PHYSICAL ACTIVITY JOURNAL

	Monday	Tuesday	Wednesday	Thursday	Friday	Saturday	Sunday
	Minutes of moderate exercise						
Lifestyle							
Structured							
	Minutes of vigorous activity						
Lifestyle							
Structured							
Total minutes							
Total steps							

My plans

Goals:

Barriers/solutions:

Affirmations:

Week of _____

 # MY HEALTHY EATING JOURNAL

	Monday	Tuesday	Wednesday	Thursday	Friday	Saturday	Sunday
Servings eaten							
Fruits and vegetables							
Grains							
Dairy and dairy alternatives							
Meat and meat alternatives							
Fats							
Sweets							
Calories per day							

My plans

Goals:

Barriers/solutions:

Affirmations:

MY PHYSICAL ACTIVITY JOURNAL

	Monday	Tuesday	Wednesday	Thursday	Friday	Saturday	Sunday
Minutes of moderate exercise							
Lifestyle							
Structured							
Minutes of vigorous activity							
Lifestyle							
Structured							
Total minutes							
Total steps							

My plans

Goals:

Barriers/solutions:

Affirmations:

Week of _____

MY HEALTHY EATING JOURNAL

	Monday	Tuesday	Wednesday	Thursday	Friday	Saturday	Sunday
				Servings eaten			
Fruits and vegetables							
Grains							
Dairy and dairy alternatives							
Meat and meat alternatives							
Fats							
Sweets							
Calories per day							

My plans

Goals:

Barriers/solutions:

Affirmations:

MY PHYSICAL ACTIVITY JOURNAL

	Monday	Tuesday	Wednesday	Thursday	Friday	Saturday	Sunday
Minutes of moderate exercise							
Lifestyle							
Structured							
Minutes of vigorous activity							
Lifestyle							
Structured							
Total minutes							
Total steps							

My plans

Goals:

Barriers/solutions:

Affirmations:

Week of _____

MY HEALTHY EATING JOURNAL

	Monday	Tuesday	Wednesday	Thursday	Friday	Saturday	Sunday
				Servings eaten			
Fruits and vegetables							
Grains							
Dairy and dairy alternatives							
Meat and meat alternatives							
Fats							
Sweets							
Calories per day							

My plans

Goals:

Barriers/solutions:

Affirmations:

MY PHYSICAL ACTIVITY JOURNAL

	Monday	Tuesday	Wednesday	Thursday	Friday	Saturday	Sunday
Minutes of moderate exercise							
Lifestyle							
Structured							
Minutes of vigorous activity							
Lifestyle							
Structured							
Total minutes							
Total steps							

My plans

Goals:

Barriers/solutions:

Affirmations:

Week of _____

MY HEALTHY EATING JOURNAL

	Monday	Tuesday	Wednesday	Thursday	Friday	Saturday	Sunday
				Servings eaten			
Fruits and vegetables							
Grains							
Dairy and dairy alternatives							
Meat and meat alternatives							
Fats							
Sweets							
Calories per day							

My plans

Goals:

Barriers/solutions:

Affirmations:

MY PHYSICAL ACTIVITY JOURNAL

	Monday	Tuesday	Wednesday	Thursday	Friday	Saturday	Sunday
Minutes of moderate exercise							
Lifestyle							
Structured							
Minutes of vigorous activity							
Lifestyle							
Structured							
Total minutes							
Total steps							

My plans

Goals:

Barriers/solutions:

Affirmations:

Week of _____

MY HEALTHY EATING JOURNAL

	Monday	Tuesday	Wednesday	Thursday	Friday	Saturday	Sunday
	Servings eaten						
Fruits and vegetables							
Grains							
Dairy and dairy alternatives							
Meat and meat alternatives							
Fats							
Sweets							
Calories per day							

My plans
Goals:
Barriers/solutions:
Affirmations:

MY PHYSICAL ACTIVITY JOURNAL

	Monday	Tuesday	Wednesday	Thursday	Friday	Saturday	Sunday
Minutes of moderate exercise							
Lifestyle							
Structured							
Minutes of vigorous activity							
Lifestyle							
Structured							
Total minutes							
Total steps							

My plans

Goals:

Barriers/solutions:

Affirmations:

Week of _____

MY HEALTHY EATING JOURNAL

	Monday	Tuesday	Wednesday	Thursday	Friday	Saturday	Sunday
				Servings eaten			
Fruits and vegetables							
Grains							
Dairy and dairy alternatives							
Meat and meat alternatives							
Fats							
Sweets							
Calories per day							

My plans

Goals:

Barriers/solutions:

Affirmations:

MY PHYSICAL ACTIVITY JOURNAL

	Monday	Tuesday	Wednesday	Thursday	Friday	Saturday	Sunday
Minutes of moderate exercise							
Lifestyle							
Structured							
Minutes of vigorous activity							
Lifestyle							
Structured							
Total minutes							
Total steps							

My plans

Goals:

Barriers/solutions:

Affirmations:

Week of _____

MY HEALTHY EATING JOURNAL

	Monday	Tuesday	Wednesday	Thursday	Friday	Saturday	Sunday
Servings eaten							
Fruits and vegetables							
Grains							
Dairy and dairy alternatives							
Meat and meat alternatives							
Fats							
Sweets							
Calories per day							

My plans

Goals:

Barriers/solutions:

Affirmations:

MY PHYSICAL ACTIVITY JOURNAL

	Monday	Tuesday	Wednesday	Thursday	Friday	Saturday	Sunday
Minutes of moderate exercise							
Lifestyle							
Structured							
Minutes of vigorous activity							
Lifestyle							
Structured							
Total minutes							
Total steps							

My plans

Goals:

Barriers/solutions:

Affirmations:

Week of _____

MY HEALTHY EATING JOURNAL

	Monday	Tuesday	Wednesday	Thursday	Friday	Saturday	Sunday
				Servings eaten			
Fruits and vegetables							
Grains							
Dairy and dairy alternatives							
Meat and meat alternatives							
Fats							
Sweets							
Calories per day							

My plans

Goals:

Barriers/solutions:

Affirmations:

MY PHYSICAL ACTIVITY JOURNAL

	Monday	Tuesday	Wednesday	Thursday	Friday	Saturday	Sunday
Minutes of moderate exercise							
Lifestyle							
Structured							
Minutes of vigorous activity							
Lifestyle							
Structured							
Total minutes							
Total steps							

My plans

Goals:

Barriers/solutions:

Affirmations:

Week of _____

 # MY HEALTHY EATING JOURNAL

	Monday	Tuesday	Wednesday	Thursday	Friday	Saturday	Sunday
	Servings eaten						
Fruits and vegetables							
Grains							
Dairy and dairy alternatives							
Meat and meat alternatives							
Fats							
Sweets							
Calories per day							

My plans
Goals:
Barriers/solutions:
Affirmations:

MY PHYSICAL ACTIVITY JOURNAL

	Monday	Tuesday	Wednesday	Thursday	Friday	Saturday	Sunday
Minutes of moderate exercise							
Lifestyle							
Structured							
Minutes of vigorous activity							
Lifestyle							
Structured							
Total minutes							
Total steps							

My plans

Goals:

Barriers/solutions:

Affirmations:

Week of _____

MY HEALTHY EATING JOURNAL

	Monday	Tuesday	Wednesday	Thursday	Friday	Saturday	Sunday
	Servings eaten						
Fruits and vegetables							
Grains							
Dairy and dairy alternatives							
Meat and meat alternatives							
Fats							
Sweets							
Calories per day							

My plans

Goals:

Barriers/solutions:

Affirmations:

MY PHYSICAL ACTIVITY JOURNAL

	Monday	Tuesday	Wednesday	Thursday	Friday	Saturday	Sunday
Minutes of moderate exercise							
Lifestyle							
Structured							
Minutes of vigorous activity							
Lifestyle							
Structured							
Total minutes							
Total steps							

My plans

Goals:

Barriers/solutions:

Affirmations:

Week of _____

MY HEALTHY EATING JOURNAL

	Monday	Tuesday	Wednesday	Thursday	Friday	Saturday	Sunday
				Servings eaten			
Fruits and vegetables							
Grains							
Dairy and dairy alternatives							
Meat and meat alternatives							
Fats							
Sweets							
Calories per day							

My plans

Goals:

Barriers/solutions:

Affirmations:

MY PHYSICAL ACTIVITY JOURNAL

	Monday	Tuesday	Wednesday	Thursday	Friday	Saturday	Sunday
Minutes of moderate exercise							
Lifestyle							
Structured							
Minutes of vigorous activity							
Lifestyle							
Structured							
Total minutes							
Total steps							

My plans

Goals:

Barriers/solutions:

Affirmations:

Week of _____

MY HEALTHY EATING JOURNAL

	Monday	Tuesday	Wednesday	Thursday	Friday	Saturday	Sunday
	Servings eaten						
Fruits and vegetables							
Grains							
Dairy and dairy alternatives							
Meat and meat alternatives							
Fats							
Sweets							
Calories per day							

My plans
Goals:
Barriers/solutions:
Affirmations:

MY PHYSICAL ACTIVITY JOURNAL

	Monday	Tuesday	Wednesday	Thursday	Friday	Saturday	Sunday
	Minutes of moderate exercise						
Lifestyle							
Structured							
	Minutes of vigorous activity						
Lifestyle							
Structured							
Total minutes							
Total steps							

My plans

Goals:

Barriers/solutions:

Affirmations:

Week of _____

MY HEALTHY EATING JOURNAL

	Monday	Tuesday	Wednesday	Thursday	Friday	Saturday	Sunday
				Servings eaten			
Fruits and vegetables							
Grains							
Dairy and dairy alternatives							
Meat and meat alternatives							
Fats							
Sweets							
Calories per day							

My plans

Goals:

Barriers/solutions:

Affirmations:

MY PHYSICAL ACTIVITY JOURNAL

	Monday	Tuesday	Wednesday	Thursday	Friday	Saturday	Sunday
Minutes of moderate exercise							
Lifestyle							
Structured							
Minutes of vigorous activity							
Lifestyle							
Structured							
Total minutes							
Total steps							

My plans

Goals:

Barriers/solutions:

Affirmations:

Week of _____

MY HEALTHY EATING JOURNAL

	Monday	Tuesday	Wednesday	Thursday	Friday	Saturday	Sunday
				Servings eaten			
Fruits and vegetables							
Grains							
Dairy and dairy alternatives							
Meat and meat alternatives							
Fats							
Sweets							
Calories per day							

My plans

Goals:

Barriers/solutions:

Affirmations:

MY PHYSICAL ACTIVITY JOURNAL

	Monday	Tuesday	Wednesday	Thursday	Friday	Saturday	Sunday
Minutes of moderate exercise							
Lifestyle							
Structured							
Minutes of vigorous activity							
Lifestyle							
Structured							
Total minutes							
Total steps							

My plans

Goals:

Barriers/solutions:

Affirmations:

Week of _____

MY HEALTHY EATING JOURNAL

	Monday	Tuesday	Wednesday	Thursday	Friday	Saturday	Sunday
Servings eaten							
Fruits and vegetables							
Grains							
Dairy and dairy alternatives							
Meat and meat alternatives							
Fats							
Sweets							
Calories per day							

My plans
Goals:
Barriers/solutions:
Affirmations:

MY PHYSICAL ACTIVITY JOURNAL

	Monday	Tuesday	Wednesday	Thursday	Friday	Saturday	Sunday
Minutes of moderate exercise							
Lifestyle							
Structured							
Minutes of vigorous activity							
Lifestyle							
Structured							
Total minutes							
Total steps							

My plans

Goals:

Barriers/solutions:

Affirmations:

Week of _____

MY HEALTHY EATING JOURNAL

	Monday	Tuesday	Wednesday	Thursday	Friday	Saturday	Sunday
				Servings eaten			
Fruits and vegetables							
Grains							
Dairy and dairy alternatives							
Meat and meat alternatives							
Fats							
Sweets							
Calories per day							

My plans
Goals:
Barriers/solutions:
Affirmations:

MY PHYSICAL ACTIVITY JOURNAL

	Monday	Tuesday	Wednesday	Thursday	Friday	Saturday	Sunday
Minutes of moderate exercise							
Lifestyle							
Structured							
Minutes of vigorous activity							
Lifestyle							
Structured							
Total minutes							
Total steps							

My plans

Goals:

Barriers/solutions:

Affirmations:

Week of _____

	Monday	Tuesday	Wednesday	Thursday	Friday	Saturday	Sunday
	Servings eaten						
Fruits and vegetables							
Grains							
Dairy and dairy alternatives							
Meat and meat alternatives							
Fats							
Sweets							
Calories per day							

My plans

Goals:

Barriers/solutions:

Affirmations:

MY PHYSICAL ACTIVITY JOURNAL

	Monday	Tuesday	Wednesday	Thursday	Friday	Saturday	Sunday
Minutes of moderate exercise							
Lifestyle							
Structured							
Minutes of vigorous activity							
Lifestyle							
Structured							
Total minutes							
Total steps							

My plans

Goals:

Barriers/solutions:

Affirmations:

Week of _____

MY HEALTHY EATING JOURNAL

	Monday	Tuesday	Wednesday	Thursday	Friday	Saturday	Sunday
				Servings eaten			
Fruits and vegetables							
Grains							
Dairy and dairy alternatives							
Meat and meat alternatives							
Fats							
Sweets							
Calories per day							

My plans

Goals:

Barriers/solutions:

Affirmations:

MY PHYSICAL ACTIVITY JOURNAL

	Monday	Tuesday	Wednesday	Thursday	Friday	Saturday	Sunday
Minutes of moderate exercise							
Lifestyle							
Structured							
Minutes of vigorous activity							
Lifestyle							
Structured							
Total minutes							
Total steps							

My plans

Goals:

Barriers/solutions:

Affirmations:

Week of _____

MY HEALTHY EATING JOURNAL

	Monday	Tuesday	Wednesday	Thursday	Friday	Saturday	Sunday
				Servings eaten			
Fruits and vegetables							
Grains							
Dairy and dairy alternatives							
Meat and meat alternatives							
Fats							
Sweets							
Calories per day							

My plans

Goals:

Barriers/solutions:

Affirmations:

MY PHYSICAL ACTIVITY JOURNAL

	Monday	Tuesday	Wednesday	Thursday	Friday	Saturday	Sunday
Minutes of moderate exercise							
Lifestyle							
Structured							
Minutes of vigorous activity							
Lifestyle							
Structured							
Total minutes							
Total steps							

My plans

Goals:

Barriers/solutions:

Affirmations:

Week of _____

MY HEALTHY EATING JOURNAL

	Monday	Tuesday	Wednesday	Thursday	Friday	Saturday	Sunday
				Servings eaten			
Fruits and vegetables							
Grains							
Dairy and dairy alternatives							
Meat and meat alternatives							
Fats							
Sweets							
Calories per day							

My plans

Goals:

Barriers/solutions:

Affirmations:

MY PHYSICAL ACTIVITY JOURNAL

	Monday	Tuesday	Wednesday	Thursday	Friday	Saturday	Sunday
Minutes of moderate exercise							
Lifestyle							
Structured							
Minutes of vigorous activity							
Lifestyle							
Structured							
Total minutes							
Total steps							

My plans

Goals:

Barriers/solutions:

Affirmations:

Week of _____

MY HEALTHY EATING JOURNAL

	Monday	Tuesday	Wednesday	Thursday	Friday	Saturday	Sunday
	Servings eaten						
Fruits and vegetables							
Grains							
Dairy and dairy alternatives							
Meat and meat alternatives							
Fats							
Sweets							
Calories per day							

My plans
Goals:
Barriers/solutions:
Affirmations:

MY PHYSICAL ACTIVITY JOURNAL

	Monday	Tuesday	Wednesday	Thursday	Friday	Saturday	Sunday
Minutes of moderate exercise							
Lifestyle							
Structured							
Minutes of vigorous activity							
Lifestyle							
Structured							
Total minutes							
Total steps							

My plans

Goals:

Barriers/solutions:

Affirmations:

MY HEALTHY EATING JOURNAL

	Monday	Tuesday	Wednesday	Thursday	Friday	Saturday	Sunday
				Servings eaten			
Fruits and vegetables							
Grains							
Dairy and dairy alternatives							
Meat and meat alternatives							
Fats							
Sweets							
Calories per day							

My plans

Goals:

Barriers/solutions:

Affirmations:

MY PHYSICAL ACTIVITY JOURNAL

	Monday	Tuesday	Wednesday	Thursday	Friday	Saturday	Sunday
Minutes of moderate exercise							
Lifestyle							
Structured							
Minutes of vigorous activity							
Lifestyle							
Structured							
Total minutes							
Total steps							

My plans

Goals:

Barriers/solutions:

Affirmations:

Week of _____

MY HEALTHY EATING JOURNAL

	Monday	Tuesday	Wednesday	Thursday	Friday	Saturday	Sunday
				Servings eaten			
Fruits and vegetables							
Grains							
Dairy and dairy alternatives							
Meat and meat alternatives							
Fats							
Sweets							
Calories per day							

My plans
Goals:
Barriers/solutions:
Affirmations:

MY PHYSICAL ACTIVITY JOURNAL

	Monday	Tuesday	Wednesday	Thursday	Friday	Saturday	Sunday
Minutes of moderate exercise							
Lifestyle							
Structured							
Minutes of vigorous activity							
Lifestyle							
Structured							
Total minutes							
Total steps							

My plans

Goals:

Barriers/solutions:

Affirmations:

Week of _____

MY HEALTHY EATING JOURNAL

	Monday	Tuesday	Wednesday	Thursday	Friday	Saturday	Sunday
				Servings eaten			
Fruits and vegetables							
Grains							
Dairy and dairy alternatives							
Meat and meat alternatives							
Fats							
Sweets							
Calories per day							

My plans

Goals:

Barriers/solutions:

Affirmations:

MY PHYSICAL ACTIVITY JOURNAL

	Monday	Tuesday	Wednesday	Thursday	Friday	Saturday	Sunday
Minutes of moderate exercise							
Lifestyle							
Structured							
Minutes of vigorous activity							
Lifestyle							
Structured							
Total minutes							
Total steps							

My plans

Goals:

Barriers/solutions:

Affirmations:

Week of _____

MY HEALTHY EATING JOURNAL

	Monday	Tuesday	Wednesday	Thursday	Friday	Saturday	Sunday
	Servings eaten						
Fruits and vegetables							
Grains							
Dairy and dairy alternatives							
Meat and meat alternatives							
Fats							
Sweets							
Calories per day							

My plans
Goals:
Barriers/solutions:
Affirmations:

MY PHYSICAL ACTIVITY JOURNAL

	Monday	Tuesday	Wednesday	Thursday	Friday	Saturday	Sunday
Minutes of moderate exercise							
Lifestyle							
Structured							
Minutes of vigorous activity							
Lifestyle							
Structured							
Total minutes							
Total steps							

My plans

Goals:

Barriers/solutions:

Affirmations:

Week of _____

MY HEALTHY EATING JOURNAL

	Monday	Tuesday	Wednesday	Thursday	Friday	Saturday	Sunday
				Servings eaten			
Fruits and vegetables							
Grains							
Dairy and dairy alternatives							
Meat and meat alternatives							
Fats							
Sweets							
Calories per day							

My plans
Goals:
Barriers/solutions:
Affirmations:

MY PHYSICAL ACTIVITY JOURNAL

	Monday	Tuesday	Wednesday	Thursday	Friday	Saturday	Sunday
Minutes of moderate exercise							
Lifestyle							
Structured							
Minutes of vigorous activity							
Lifestyle							
Structured							
Total minutes							
Total steps							

My plans

Goals:

Barriers/solutions:

Affirmations:

Week of _____

MY HEALTHY EATING JOURNAL

	Monday	Tuesday	Wednesday	Thursday	Friday	Saturday	Sunday
	Servings eaten						
Fruits and vegetables							
Grains							
Dairy and dairy alternatives							
Meat and meat alternatives							
Fats							
Sweets							
Calories per day							

My plans
Goals:
Barriers/solutions:
Affirmations:

MY PHYSICAL ACTIVITY JOURNAL

	Monday	Tuesday	Wednesday	Thursday	Friday	Saturday	Sunday
Minutes of moderate exercise							
Lifestyle							
Structured							
Minutes of vigorous activity							
Lifestyle							
Structured							
Total minutes							
Total steps							

My plans

Goals:

Barriers/solutions:

Affirmations:

Week of _____

MY HEALTHY EATING JOURNAL

	Monday	Tuesday	Wednesday	Thursday	Friday	Saturday	Sunday
				Servings eaten			
Fruits and vegetables							
Grains							
Dairy and dairy alternatives							
Meat and meat alternatives							
Fats							
Sweets							
Calories per day							

My plans
Goals:
Barriers/solutions:
Affirmations:

MY PHYSICAL ACTIVITY JOURNAL

	Monday	Tuesday	Wednesday	Thursday	Friday	Saturday	Sunday
Minutes of moderate exercise							
Lifestyle							
Structured							
Minutes of vigorous activity							
Lifestyle							
Structured							
Total minutes							
Total steps							

My plans

Goals:

Barriers/solutions:

Affirmations:

Week of _____

MY HEALTHY EATING JOURNAL

	Monday	Tuesday	Wednesday	Thursday	Friday	Saturday	Sunday
				Servings eaten			
Fruits and vegetables							
Grains							
Dairy and dairy alternatives							
Meat and meat alternatives							
Fats							
Sweets							
Calories per day							

My plans

Goals:

Barriers/solutions:

Affirmations:

MY PHYSICAL ACTIVITY JOURNAL

	Monday	Tuesday	Wednesday	Thursday	Friday	Saturday	Sunday
Minutes of moderate exercise							
Lifestyle							
Structured							
Minutes of vigorous activity							
Lifestyle							
Structured							
Total minutes							
Total steps							

My plans

Goals:

Barriers/solutions:

Affirmations:

Week of _____

MY HEALTHY EATING JOURNAL

	Monday	Tuesday	Wednesday	Thursday	Friday	Saturday	Sunday
Servings eaten							
Fruits and vegetables							
Grains							
Dairy and dairy alternatives							
Meat and meat alternatives							
Fats							
Sweets							
Calories per day							

My plans

Goals:

Barriers/solutions:

Affirmations:

MY PHYSICAL ACTIVITY JOURNAL

	Monday	Tuesday	Wednesday	Thursday	Friday	Saturday	Sunday
Minutes of moderate exercise							
Lifestyle							
Structured							
Minutes of vigorous activity							
Lifestyle							
Structured							
Total minutes							
Total steps							

My plans

Goals:

Barriers/solutions:

Affirmations:

Week of _____

MY HEALTHY EATING JOURNAL

	Monday	Tuesday	Wednesday	Thursday	Friday	Saturday	Sunday
	Servings eaten						
Fruits and vegetables							
Grains							
Dairy and dairy alternatives							
Meat and meat alternatives							
Fats							
Sweets							
Calories per day							

My plans
Goals:
Barriers/solutions:
Affirmations:

MY PHYSICAL ACTIVITY JOURNAL

	Monday	Tuesday	Wednesday	Thursday	Friday	Saturday	Sunday
	Minutes of moderate exercise						
Lifestyle							
Structured							
	Minutes of vigorous activity						
Lifestyle							
Structured							
Total minutes							
Total steps							

My plans

Goals:

Barriers/solutions:

Affirmations:

APPENDIX A

GUIDELINES FOR MODERATE-INTENSITY PHYSICAL ACTIVITY

Moderate-intensity activity can be defined as activity that is equivalent to a brisk walk. That means walking 3 to 4 miles per hour (4.8 to 6.4 kilometers), or walking 1 mile (1.6 kilometers) in 15 to 20 minutes. How does this compare to light or vigorous activity? If you are strolling through the park or walking while window shopping, you are probably walking at a light pace. If you are walking with a purpose, for instance to catch a bus or get to a meeting you're a little late for, you are probably walking at a moderate pace. If you are walking very quickly (for instance, doing aerobic fitness walking), your heart rate goes up and you breathe harder, so you are probably walking at a vigorous pace.

Besides walking, there are many activities that are moderately intense. A few examples are social dancing, mowing the lawn with a motorized push mower, or taking a low-impact aerobics class. For more examples, see appendix C on page 150.

Moderate-intensity activity has been shown to significantly improve health if done regularly. To improve your health with moderate-intensity activity, be sure to accumulate at least 30 minutes a day (you can do this in shorter bouts, such as three bouts of 10 minutes each) on at least five days each week.

U.S. Surgeon General's Statement on Physical Activity and Health

All Americans should engage in regular physical activity at a level appropriate to their capabilities, needs, and interests. Significant health benefits can be obtained by setting and reaching a goal of accumulating at least 30 minutes of moderate-intensity physical activity on most, preferably all, days of the week. Those who currently meet these standards may derive additional benefits by becoming more physically active or including vigorous activity.

U.S. Department of Health and Human Services. 1996. *Physical activity and health: A report of the surgeon general.* Atlanta: U.S. Department of Health and Human Services, Centers for Disease Control and Prevention, National Center for Chronic Disease Prevention and Health Promotion. Available at www.cdc.gov/nccdphp/sgr/sgr.htm.

Adapted from Human Kinetics, 2002, *ALED facilitator guide* (Champaign, IL: Human Kinetics), 3.

APPENDIX B

GUIDELINES FOR VIGOROUS-INTENSITY PHYSICAL ACTIVITY

Agencies such as the American College of Sports Medicine (ACSM) have developed reliable guidelines on engaging in vigorous activities such as running, aerobics, and strength training. The following outlines these guidelines:

GUIDELINES FOR AEROBIC ACTIVITY

These guidelines are appropriate for any kind of endurance activities such as running, swimming laps, or doing aerobics.

* Do aerobic activity 3 to 5 times per week.

* Warm up gradually 5 to 10 minutes before your aerobic activity.

* Maintain your aerobic intensity for 20 to 60 minutes of continuous or intermittent (minimum of 10-minute bouts) of activity accumulated throughout the day.

* Gradually decrease intensity, then stretch to maintain flexibility.

* If weight loss is a major goal, participate in aerobic activity at least 30 minutes 5 days per week.

* On days when you cannot complete your entire program, complete whatever portion you can, even if it's only 10 or 15 minutes. In addition, make a point to do more lifestyle physical activity throughout the day. Remember that all appropriate physical activity contributes to your overall health. Don't try to make up sessions by cramming them all into a single weekend, by increasing the length of a single session, or by increasing the intensity of a session. If you do this, you will increase your risk of injury.

DETERMINING INTENSITY FOR AEROBIC ACTIVITIES

One good way to measure the intensity of your aerobic activity is to measure your heart rate. The ACSM has determined that exercising in what is known as your target heart rate range will maximize the good effects of the activity and will minimize the risk of injury. Your target heart rate range is 60 to 90% of your estimated maximal heart rate. The following shows you how to calculate your range:

1. Estimate your maximal heart rate using this formula:

   220 – ___ (your age) = ___(estimated maximal heart rate)

2. Determine the lower end of your target heart range by multiplying your maximal heart rate by 0.6:

   ___(your maximal heart rate) $\times$ 0.6 = ___(low end of target heart rate range)

3. Determine the upper end of your target heart rate range by multiplying your estimated maximum heart rate by 0.9:

   ___(your maximal heart rate) $\times$ 0.9 = ___(high end of your target heart rate range)

4. Your target heart rate range is 60 to 90% of your maximal heart rate.

   My target heart rate range is ___(60% of maximum) to ___(90% of maximum).

Within this range, select an intensity that is comfortable for you. If you are new to vigorous activity, don't start with too high an intensity; you can always increase intensity later when you are more comfortable with this type of activity.

Be aware that some medications (such as blood pressure medications) may affect your heart rate during physical activity. If you are taking any of these medications, this method of measuring intensity may not work. See your doctor before determining your appropriate intensity of vigorous activity.

GUIDELINES FOR MUSCULAR FITNESS ACTIVITIES

Muscular fitness activities (also known as strength training) are a great way to increase strength, maintain or improve bone density, and control weight. You can do these exercises in several different ways, including using strength training equipment, hand weights, and resistance bands. The American College of Sports Medicine has issued the following guidelines for improving muscular fitness:

* Include exercises for all the major muscle groups in both the upper and lower body.

* Complete 8 to 15 repetitions of each exercise. When you can easily complete 15 repetitions, increase workload in one of two ways: Increase the amount of resistance or weight, or do a second set of 8 to 15 repetitions.

* Participate in muscular fitness activities for all major muscle groups 2 or 3 times a week. Allow a rest period of at least 48 hours between sessions.

References

American College of Sports Medicine. 2003. *ACSM fitness book.* (Champaign, IL: Human Kinetics), pp 160-163.

APPENDIX C

EXAMPLES OF LIGHT, MODERATE, AND VIGOROUS ACTIVITIES

One of the great things about physical activity is that, with so many different options, you are sure to find something you enjoy. The following is a list of some common activities of moderate and vigorous intensity. Both lifestyle and structured activities are included.

You'll also find light activities listed here. These are not intense enough to significantly improve health, but we've included them for reference purposes. One way to increase your physical activity is to find ways to boost the intensity of light activities you already do in order to make them moderate or vigorous. Approximate conversions from miles to kilometers follow.

1 mile = 1.6 kilometers

2 miles = 3.2 kilometers

3 miles = 4.8 kilometers

4 miles = 6.4 kilometers

4.5 miles = 7.2 kilometers

5 miles = 8 kilometers

6 miles = 9.7 kilometers

7 miles = 11.3 kilometers

8 miles = 12.9 kilometers

9 miles = 14.5 kilometers

10 miles = 16 kilometers

References

Ainsworth, B.E., Haskell, W.L., Leon, A.S., et. al. 1993. "Compendium of physical activities: Classification of energy costs of human physical activities." *Medicine and Science in Sports and Exercise* 25(1): 71 – 80.

U.S. Department of Health and Human Services. 1999. *Promoting physical activity: A guide for community action.* Champaign, IL: Human Kinetics.

Light-intensity activities (use fewer than 3.5 calories/min)	Moderate-intensity activities (use 3.5-7 calories/min)	Vigorous-intensity activities (use more than 7 calories/min)
Walking casually (less than 3 mph), strolling, window shopping	Walking briskly (3-4.5 mph), hiking	Racewalking or aerobic walking (5 mph or faster), jogging, running, backpacking
Bicycling less than 5 mph, stationary bicycling (light effort)	Bicycling (5-9 mph), stationary bicycling (moderate effort)	Bicycling more than 10 mph or on steep hill, stationary bicycling (hard effort)
Floating in water	Recreational swimming, water aerobics	Swimming laps, water jogging
Stretching exercises	Calisthenics (light), yoga, using stair climber (light to moderate pace), weight training and bodybuilding, aerobic dance (low impact)	Vigorous calisthenics (e.g., push-ups, pull-ups), martial arts, jumping rope, using stair climber (fast pace), circuit weight training, aerobic dance (high impact), step aerobics
Slow ballroom dancing	Dancing (e.g., ballroom, line, square, folk, modern, ballet, disco)	Professional or competitive ballroom dancing, clogging
Golf (riding in a cart)	Golf (carrying clubs)	
Light housework (e.g., dusting, sweeping, making beds)	Moderate housework (e.g., scrubbing floors, washing windows, moving light furniture, carrying heavy bags of trash)	Heavy housework (e.g., moving heavy furniture, carrying household items weighing 25 lb [11 kg] or more up stairs)
Light gardening or yard work (e.g., weeding while sitting, watering lawn, mowing lawn on riding mower)	Moderate gardening or yard work (e.g., raking lawn, mowing lawn with motorized push mower, weeding while standing or bending)	Heavy gardening or yard work (shoveling snow, mowing lawn with motorized push mower, digging ditches)
Sitting and playing with children (e.g., board games, reading, computer, TV)	Actively playing with children (e.g., walking, running, chasing, shooting baskets)	Vigorously playing with children (e.g., running long distances or playing strenuous games), racewalking or jogging while pushing a stroller
Light occupational work (computer work, talking on phone, standing, driving)	Occupational work requiring extended periods of walking, moving objects weighing less than 75 lb [34 kg] (e.g., maid service, waiting tables)	Occupational work requiring extended periods of running, moving objects 75 lb [34 kg] or heavier (e.g., fitness instructing, firefighting, heavy construction)

Adapted, by permission, from B.E. Ainsworth, W.L. Haskell, A.S. Leon, et al., 1993, "Compendium of physical activities: Classification of energy costs of human physical activities," *Medicine and Science in Sports and Exercise* 25(1): 71-80.

APPENDIX D

WHAT IS A SERVING?

People often confuse portions with serving sizes. A portion is how much food you actually are served or eat. A serving is the amount of a given food determined by health experts to be an appropriate amount for a person to eat. These are the amounts used to make national recommendations. Confusing portion with serving can lead to overeating. For instance, a *portion* of pasta served to you in a restaurant may actually be four to six *servings* of the bread group.

The sizes of common packaged foods such as soda and snack foods and portion sizes in restaurants have increased dramatically since the 1970s. By staying aware of the recommended serving sizes, you will be much more likely to keep your weight under control and to eat a healthy diet.

The following describes serving sizes of common foods in two ways. First you will find the measured amount or weight of food in a serving. For instance, a serving of pasta is ½ cup. But you can't always measure your food, so we've also listed some visual cues you can use. A visual cue for a 1/2-cup serving of pasta is a computer mouse; they are about the same size.

References

Carpenter, Ruth and Carrie Finley. 2005. *Healthy eating every day.* (Champaign, IL: Human Kinetics), pp. 10-11, 88-89, 102.

Type of food	Serving size (1 serving)	Visual cue
Bread, cereal, rice, pasta, potatoes, corn		
Rice, pasta, cooked cereal, or corn	1/2 cup (80 g) rice 1/2 cup (70 g) pasta 1/2 cup (80 g) corn 1/2 cup (120 g) cooked cereal	Small computer mouse
Ready-to-eat cereal	1 cup (30 g)	Tennis ball
Bagel	1 small bagel (1/2 large bagel)	Hockey puck
Bread	1 slice	Stack of 3 computer disks
Roll or muffin	1 small roll or muffin	Plum
Fruits and vegetables		
Apple, orange, peach	Medium whole piece	Baseball
Dried fruit (e.g., raisins)	1/4 cup (40 g)	Golf ball
Fruit juice	3/4 cup (180 ml)	
Leafy greens (e.g., lettuce, raw spinach)	1 cup (55 g)	1/2 of a grapefruit
Cooked vegetables	1/2 cup (85 g)	Small computer mouse
Dairy and dairy alternatives		
Milk or yogurt	1 cup (240 ml)	Small (8 oz or 240 ml) milk carton
Soy milk or yogurt	1 cup (240 ml)	Small (8 oz or 240 ml) milk carton
Firm cheese (e.g., Cheddar)	1-1/2 oz (45 g)	6 dice
Soft cheese (e.g., cottage)	1/2 cup (85 g)	Small computer mouse
Meat and meat alternatives		
Meat, poultry fish, cooked	2-3 oz (60-85 g)	Deck of playing cards
Legumes, cooked (e.g., kidney beans)	1 cup	Tennis ball
Peanut butter	2 Tbsp (30 ml)	Roll of film
Tofu, cooked	1/2 cup (90 g)	Computer mouse

Adapted, by permission, from R. Carpenter and C. Finley, 2005. *Healthy eating every day.* (Champaign, IL: Human Kinetics), p. 89.

APPENDIX E

Physical Activity Readiness
Questionnaire - PAR-Q
(revised 2002)

PAR-Q & YOU

(A Questionnaire for People Aged 15 to 69)

Regular physical activity is fun and healthy, and increasingly more people are starting to become more active every day. Being more active is very safe for most people. However, some people should check with their doctor before they start becoming much more physically active.

If you are planning to become much more physically active than you are now, start by answering the seven questions in the box below. If you are between the ages of 15 and 69, the PAR-Q will tell you if you should check with your doctor before you start. If you are over 69 years of age, and you are not used to being very active, check with your doctor.

Common sense is your best guide when you answer these questions. Please read the questions carefully and answer each one honestly: check YES or NO.

YES	NO		
☐	☐	1.	Has your doctor ever said that you have a heart condition <u>and</u> that you should only do physical activity recommended by a doctor?
☐	☐	2.	Do you feel pain in your chest when you do physical activity?
☐	☐	3.	In the past month, have you had chest pain when you were not doing physical activity?
☐	☐	4.	Do you lose your balance because of dizziness or do you ever lose consciousness?
☐	☐	5.	Do you have a bone or joint problem (for example, back, knee or hip) that could be made worse by a change in your physical activity?
☐	☐	6.	Is your doctor currently prescribing drugs (for example, water pills) for your blood pressure or heart condition?
☐	☐	7.	Do you know of <u>any other reason</u> why you should not do physical activity?

If

you

answered

YES to one or more questions

Talk with your doctor by phone or in person BEFORE you start becoming much more physically active or BEFORE you have a fitness appraisal. Tell your doctor about the PAR-Q and which questions you answered YES.

- You may be able to do any activity you want — as long as you start slowly and build up gradually. Or, you may need to restrict your activities to those which are safe for you. Talk with your doctor about the kinds of activities you wish to participate in and follow his/her advice.
- Find out which community programs are safe and helpful for you.

NO to all questions

If you answered NO honestly to <u>all</u> PAR-Q questions, you can be reasonably sure that you can:
- start becoming much more physically active – begin slowly and build up gradually. This is the safest and easiest way to go.
- take part in a fitness appraisal – this is an excellent way to determine your basic fitness so that you can plan the best way for you to live actively. It is also highly recommended that you have your blood pressure evaluated. If your reading is over 144/94, talk with your doctor before you start becoming much more physically active.

DELAY BECOMING MUCH MORE ACTIVE:
- if you are not feeling well because of a temporary illness such as a cold or a fever – wait until you feel better; or
- if you are or may be pregnant – talk to your doctor before you start becoming more active.

PLEASE NOTE: If your health changes so that you then answer YES to any of the above questions, tell your fitness or health professional. Ask whether you should change your physical activity plan.

<u>Informed Use of the PAR-Q:</u> The Canadian Society for Exercise Physiology, Health Canada, and their agents assume no liability for persons who undertake physical activity, and if in doubt after completing this questionnaire, consult your doctor prior to physical activity.

No changes permitted. You are encouraged to photocopy the PAR-Q but only if you use the entire form.

NOTE: If the PAR-Q is being given to a person before he or she participates in a physical activity program or a fitness appraisal, this section may be used for legal or administrative purposes.

"I have read, understood and completed this questionnaire. Any questions I had were answered to my full satisfaction."

NAME _____

SIGNATURE _____ DATE _____

SIGNATURE OF PARENT _____ WITNESS _____
or GUARDIAN (for participants under the age of majority)

Note: This physical activity clearance is valid for a maximum of 12 months from the date it is completed and becomes invalid if your condition changes so that you would answer YES to any of the seven questions.

CSEP
SCPE © Canadian Society for Exercise Physiology Supported by: [🍁] Health Santé
Canada Canada

Source: Physical Activity Readiness Questionnaire (PAR-Q) © 2002. Reprinted with permission of the Canadian Society for Exercise Physiology, Inc. http://www.csep.ca/forms.asp

APPENDIX F

GUIDELINES FOR STEPS PER DAY

One way to track the amount of physical activity you get is by keeping count of the number of steps you take per day by using a step counter. Step counters are worn over the hipbone attached to a belt or the waistband of your clothes and can be purchased at sports equipment stores or directly from the manufacturers. The following discussion answers the most frequently asked questions in regards to step counters.

1. **How do I know how many steps I take?** Before you can set a goal for steps per day, it's good to know how many steps you normally take. Wear your step counter for at least three days—preferably two weekdays and one weekend day. Put the step counter on as soon as you get up in the morning and leave it on until you go to bed at night. At the end of the day record the number of steps on the journal section of this book. By doing this you'll know your starting point. Don't forget to reset the step counter to zero before putting it on the next day.

2. **How many steps should I take each day?** If you get 10,000 or more steps per day, you are most likely meeting the public health guidelines for physical activity. Taking this number of steps is similar to accumulating 30 minutes of moderate intensity activity.

3. **That seems like a lot of steps. What if I'm not taking that many steps?** Don't worry, attaining 10,000 steps per day is easier than it might sound. To start with, most inactive people get between 2,400 and 4,000 steps just in the course of their daily living. Once you've determined how many steps you get by wearing your step counter for a few days, set a short-term goal to increase that amount by about 250–500 steps per day. For instance, if you find that you normally take 4,500 steps per day, set a goal to average 4,750–5,000 steps per day. Once you reach that goal, increase the goal another 250–500 steps per day, and so on. Consider 10,000 steps a day as a long-term goal, not something you need to accomplish immediately.

4. **How do I learn more about this?** For more information on tracking steps per day or on how to purchase a step counter see the following resources.

References

Steps to Better Health. The Cooper Institute. 2003.

Accusplit (manufactures step counters): (800) 935-1996, www.accusplit.com.

APPENDIX G

ASSESSMENT OF BODY MASS INDEX

Body mass index (BMI) measures the ratio of your weight to height and is a commonly accepted method for determining whether your weight is healthy. Calculating BMI is easy. Use the chart on page 157. Find your height across the top and your weight on the left side of the chart. (If you use the metric system, find your height across the bottom and your weight on the right side of the chart.) The point where your height and weight meet on the chart is an estimate of your BMI.

The World Health Organization has classified BMI values into these categories:

* BMI less than 18.5: underweight
* BMI between 18.5 and 24.9: normal weight
* BMI between 25 and 29.9: overweight
* BMI of 30 or greater: obese

Research has shown that a BMI of 25 or greater is associated with increased risk for chronic diseases such as heart disease, diabetes, and even some types of cancer. Knowing which category you fit into may help you better understand your overall health status and therefore help you make decisions about changing your lifestyle.

References

Carpenter, R.A. and C.E. Finley. 2005. *Healthy eating every day.* (Champaign, IL: Human Kinetics), pp. 164-165.

Adapted, by permission, from R. Carpenter and C. Finley, 2005. *Healthy eating every day.* (Champaign, IL: Human Kinetics), p. 164. Data from NIH/NHLBI. 1998. Clinical guidelines on the identification, evaluation and treatment of overweight and obesity in adults. The evidence report. National Institutes of Health. *Obesity Research* 6(suppl. 2): 51S-209S.

Body Mass Index

Height in inches

Wt. (lb)	48	49	50	51	52	53	54	55	56	57	58	59	60	61	62	63	64	65	66	67	68	69	70	71	72	73	74	75	76	77	78	Wt. (kg)
100	30.6	29.3	28.2	27.1	26.1	25.1	24.2	23.3	22.5	21.7	20.9	20.2	19.6	18.9	18.3	17.8	17.2	16.7	16.2	15.7	15.2	14.8	14.4	14.0	13.6	13.2	12.9	12.5	12.2	11.9	11.6	45.5
105	32.1	30.8	29.6	28.4	27.4	26.3	25.4	24.5	23.6	22.8	22.0	21.3	20.5	19.9	19.2	18.6	18.1	17.5	17.0	16.5	16.0	15.5	15.1	14.7	14.3	13.9	13.5	13.2	12.8	12.5	12.2	47.7
110	33.6	32.3	31.0	29.8	28.7	27.6	26.6	25.6	24.7	23.9	23.0	22.3	21.5	20.8	20.2	19.5	18.9	18.3	17.8	17.3	16.8	16.3	15.8	15.4	14.9	14.5	14.2	13.8	13.4	13.1	12.7	50.0
115	35.2	33.7	32.4	31.2	30.0	28.8	27.8	26.8	25.8	24.9	24.1	23.3	22.5	21.8	21.1	20.4	19.8	19.2	18.6	18.0	17.5	17.0	16.5	16.1	15.6	15.2	14.8	14.4	14.0	13.7	13.3	52.3
120	36.7	35.2	33.8	32.5	31.2	30.1	29.0	27.9	27.0	26.0	25.1	24.3	23.5	22.7	22.0	21.3	20.6	20.0	19.4	18.8	18.3	17.8	17.3	16.8	16.3	15.9	15.4	15.0	14.6	14.3	13.9	54.5
125	38.2	36.7	35.2	33.9	32.6	31.4	30.2	29.1	28.1	27.1	26.2	25.3	24.5	23.7	22.9	22.2	21.5	20.8	20.2	19.6	19.0	18.5	18.0	17.5	17.0	16.5	16.1	15.7	15.2	14.9	14.5	56.8
130	39.8	38.1	36.6	35.2	33.9	32.6	31.4	30.3	29.2	28.2	27.2	26.3	25.4	24.6	23.8	23.1	22.4	21.7	21.0	20.4	19.8	19.2	18.7	18.2	17.7	17.2	16.7	16.3	15.9	15.4	15.1	59.1
135	41.3	39.6	38.0	36.6	35.2	33.9	32.6	31.4	30.3	29.3	28.3	27.3	26.4	25.6	24.7	24.0	23.2	22.5	21.8	21.2	20.6	20.0	19.4	18.9	18.3	17.8	17.4	16.9	16.5	16.1	15.6	61.4
140	42.8	41.1	39.5	37.9	36.5	35.1	33.8	32.6	31.5	30.4	29.3	28.3	27.4	26.5	25.7	24.7	24.0	23.3	22.6	21.9	21.3	20.7	20.1	19.6	19.0	18.5	18.0	17.5	17.1	16.6	16.2	63.6
145	44.3	42.5	40.9	39.3	37.8	36.4	35.0	33.8	32.6	31.4	30.4	29.3	28.4	27.5	26.6	25.7	24.9	24.2	23.5	22.8	22.1	21.5	20.8	20.3	19.7	19.2	18.7	18.2	17.7	17.2	16.8	65.9
150	45.9	44.0	42.3	40.6	39.1	37.6	36.2	34.9	33.7	32.6	31.4	30.4	29.3	28.4	27.5	26.6	25.8	25.0	24.3	23.5	22.9	22.2	21.6	21.0	20.3	19.8	19.3	18.8	18.3	17.8	17.4	68.2
155	47.4	45.5	43.7	42.0	40.4	38.9	37.5	36.1	34.9	33.7	32.5	31.4	30.3	29.4	28.4	27.5	26.7	25.8	25.0	24.3	23.6	22.9	22.3	21.7	21.1	20.5	19.9	19.4	18.9	18.4	17.9	70.5
160	48.9	47.0	45.1	43.3	41.7	40.1	38.7	37.3	35.8	34.7	33.6	32.4	31.3	30.3	29.3	28.4	27.5	26.7	25.9	25.1	24.4	23.7	23.0	22.4	21.7	21.2	20.6	20.0	19.5	19.0	18.5	72.7
165	50.5	48.4	46.5	44.7	43.0	41.4	39.9	38.4	37.1	35.8	34.6	33.5	32.3	31.3	30.2	29.3	28.4	27.5	26.7	25.9	25.1	24.4	23.7	23.1	22.4	21.8	21.2	20.7	20.1	19.6	19.1	75.0
170	52.0	49.9	47.9	46.0	44.3	42.6	41.1	39.6	38.2	36.9	35.6	34.4	33.3	32.2	31.2	30.2	29.2	28.3	27.5	26.6	25.9	25.2	24.4	23.8	23.1	22.5	21.9	21.3	20.7	20.2	19.7	77.3
175	53.5	51.4	49.3	47.4	45.6	43.9	42.3	40.8	39.3	37.9	36.7	35.4	34.2	33.1	32.1	31.1	30.1	29.2	28.3	27.3	26.7	25.9	25.2	24.5	23.8	23.1	22.5	21.9	21.3	20.8	20.3	79.5
180	55.0	52.8	50.7	48.8	46.9	45.1	43.5	41.9	40.4	39.0	37.7	36.4	35.2	34.1	33.0	32.0	31.0	30.0	29.1	28.3	27.4	26.6	25.9	25.2	24.5	23.8	23.2	22.5	22.0	21.4	20.8	81.8
185	56.6	54.3	52.1	50.1	48.2	46.4	44.7	43.1	41.6	40.1	38.7	37.4	36.2	35.0	33.9	32.8	31.8	30.8	29.9	29.0	28.2	27.4	26.6	25.9	25.1	24.5	23.8	23.2	22.6	22.0	21.4	84.1
190	58.1	55.8	53.5	51.5	49.5	47.7	45.9	44.3	42.7	41.2	39.8	38.5	37.2	36.0	34.8	33.7	32.7	31.7	30.7	29.8	29.0	28.1	27.3	26.6	25.8	25.1	24.4	23.8	23.2	22.6	22.0	86.4
195	59.6	57.2	55.0	52.8	50.8	48.9	47.1	45.4	43.8	42.3	40.8	39.5	38.2	37.0	35.7	34.6	33.5	32.5	31.5	30.6	29.7	28.9	28.0	27.3	26.5	25.8	25.1	24.4	23.8	23.2	22.6	88.6
200	61.2	58.7	56.4	54.2	52.1	50.2	48.3	46.6	44.9	43.4	41.9	40.5	39.1	37.9	36.7	35.5	34.4	33.4	32.3	31.4	30.5	29.6	28.8	28.0	27.3	26.4	25.7	25.1	24.4	23.8	23.2	90.9
205	62.7	60.2	57.8	55.5	53.4	51.4	49.5	47.7	46.1	44.5	42.9	41.5	40.1	38.8	37.6	36.4	35.3	34.2	33.2	32.2	31.2	30.3	29.5	28.7	27.9	27.1	26.4	25.7	25.0	24.4	23.7	93.2
210	64.2	61.6	59.2	56.9	54.7	52.7	50.7	48.9	47.2	45.5	44.0	42.5	41.1	39.8	38.5	37.3	36.1	35.0	34.0	33.0	32.0	31.1	30.2	29.4	28.5	27.8	27.0	26.3	25.6	25.0	24.3	95.5
215	65.7	63.1	60.6	58.2	56.0	53.9	51.9	50.1	48.3	46.6	45.0	43.5	42.1	40.7	39.4	38.2	37.0	35.9	34.8	33.8	32.8	31.8	30.9	30.0	29.2	28.4	27.6	26.9	26.2	25.5	24.9	97.7
220	67.3	64.6	62.0	59.6	57.3	55.2	53.2	51.2	49.4	47.7	46.1	44.5	43.1	41.7	40.3	39.1	37.8	36.7	35.6	34.5	33.5	32.6	31.6	30.7	29.9	29.1	28.3	27.6	26.8	26.1	25.5	100.0
225	68.8	66.0	63.4	60.9	58.6	56.4	54.4	52.4	50.5	48.8	47.1	45.6	44.0	42.6	41.2	39.9	38.7	37.5	36.4	35.3	34.3	33.3	32.4	31.4	30.6	29.7	28.9	28.2	27.4	26.7	26.1	102.3
230	70.3	67.5	64.8	62.3	59.9	57.7	55.6	53.6	51.7	49.9	48.2	46.6	45.0	43.6	42.2	40.8	39.6	38.4	37.2	36.1	35.0	34.0	33.1	32.1	31.3	30.4	29.6	28.8	28.1	27.3	26.6	104.5
235	71.9	69.0	66.2	63.7	61.2	58.9	56.8	54.7	52.8	51.0	49.2	47.6	46.0	44.5	43.1	41.7	40.4	39.1	38.0	36.9	35.8	34.8	33.8	32.8	31.9	31.1	30.2	29.4	28.7	27.9	27.2	106.8
240	73.4	70.4	67.6	65.0	62.5	60.2	58.0	55.9	53.9	52.1	50.3	48.6	47.0	45.4	44.0	42.6	41.3	40.0	38.8	37.7	36.6	35.5	34.5	33.5	32.6	31.7	30.9	30.1	29.3	28.5	27.8	109.1
245	74.9	71.9	69.0	66.4	63.8	61.5	59.2	57.1	55.0	53.1	51.3	49.6	47.9	46.4	44.9	43.5	42.1	40.9	39.6	38.5	37.3	36.3	35.2	34.2	33.2	32.4	31.5	30.7	29.9	29.1	28.4	111.4
250	76.4	73.4	70.5	67.7	65.1	62.7	60.4	58.2	56.2	54.2	52.4	50.6	48.9	47.3	45.8	44.4	43.0	41.7	40.4	39.2	38.1	37.0	35.9	34.9	34.0	33.1	32.2	31.3	30.5	29.7	29.0	113.6
	1.22	1.24	1.27	1.30	1.32	1.35	1.37	1.40	1.42	1.45	1.47	1.50	1.52	1.55	1.57	1.60	1.63	1.65	1.68	1.70	1.73	1.75	1.78	1.80	1.83	1.85	1.88	1.91	1.93	1.96	1.98	

Height in meters

Key

Obese	Overweight	Normal weight	Underweight

Adapted, by permission, from J. Morrow, et al., 2005, *Measurement and evaluation in human performance*, 3rd ed. (Champaign, IL: Human Kinetics), 242-243.

ADDITIONAL RESOURCES

First Steps: Your Healthy Living Journal is meant to get you started on your way to moving more and eating better. Reading about the four steps to healthy behavior change and using the journal may inspire you to learn and do more. The following are sources of reliable information.

ACSM Fitness Book, Third Edition (Human Kinetics 2004). This book gives you the tools you need to establish an effective structure exercise program. Topics include: fitness assessment, guidelines for effective exercise, motivational tips, demonstrations of specific exercises, and an easy to follow step-by step program.

Active Living Every Day by Steven N. Blair, Andrea L. Dunn, Bess H. Marcus, Ruth Ann Carpenter, Peter E. Jaret (Human Kinetics 2001). Become and stay physically active for a lifetime with *Active Living Every Day*. This book and optional course helps you overcome your barriers to physical activity, find time to fit activity into your busy life, and discover activities that you will enjoy.

American Dietetic Association's Pocket Supermarket Guide, Third Edition by the American Dietetic Association. This book helps consumers make smart food choices based on personal dietary needs. Reflects consumer shopping trends and packed with nutrition information and shopping tips. www.eatright.org.

American Dietary Association Complete Food and Nutrition Guide, Second Edition by R.L. Duyff (John Wiley & Sons 2002). This consumer reference provides comprehensive nutrition information, including current guidelines, up-to-date research and facts, and practical tips.

calorie-count.com. This Web site lists the calorie counts for thousands of food and is a good resource for people trying to lose weight who want to keep track of calories.

Eating On the Run, Third Edition by Evelyn Tribole (Human Kinetics 2004). A terrific resource for busy people. Excellent and practical advice on how to eat healthfully at work, at home, when dining out or traveling—any time when time is limited.

Healthy Eating Every Day by Ruth Ann Carpenter, Carrie E. Finley, and The Cooper Institute (Human Kinetics 2005). Change your eating habits one bite at a time with *Healthy Eating Every Day*. This book and optional course empower you to make permanent improvements in your eating habits.

Nancy Clark's Sport Nutrition Guidebook, Third Edition by Nancy Clark (Human Kinetics 2003). The ultimate eating and nutrition resource for the physically active person. Topics include: information on how to fuel an active lifestyle, achieve a desired weight, how to eat before and after games, training sessions and competitions, information on supplements, customized eating plans and recipes.

ABOUT THE AUTHORS

Active Living Partners, a division of Human Kinetics, produces educational programs and tools that address physical inactivity and unbalanced eating—two leading causes of obesity, heart disease, and other chronic ailments. These programs, Active Living Every Day and Healthy Eating Every Day, have been successfully implemented worldwide in worksites, hospitals, community health programs, senior residences, colleges and universities, and fitness centers, as well as by individuals.

The success of Active Living programs in empowering people to permanently change their health habits can be traced to the following features:

* Focus on behavioral change. The underlying causes of poor health habits are addressed with an emphasis on lifestyle-management skills and realistically paced change.

* Scientific basis. Developed in partnership with The Cooper Institute, Active Living programs use curriculums that have been proven effective in clinical trials.

* Personalized approach. Programs may be tailored to each person's stage of readiness to change, lifestyle, and personal preferences.

* Flexible delivery options. Courses may be delivered in groups, online, or via phone or face-to-face coaching.

* Ongoing support. Comprehensive support is provided through the Active Living staff and Web site, www.ActiveLiving.info.

For more information about Active Living Partners programs, please contact Michelle Osborne at:

Active Living Partners
P.O. Box 5076
Champaign, IL 61825-5076
Phone: 800-747-4457 ext 2522
E-mail: michelleo@hkusa.com

ABOUT THE WRITERS

Maggie Spilner is the former walking columnist of *Prevention* magazine and author of three other books on walking for health and fitness. A certified trainer and registered yoga instructor, she is the founder of Walk For All Seasons, LLC, a company that organizes walking vacations and rallies.

Michele Guerra, MS, CHES, is the director of Active Living Partners at Human Kinetics. A health and fitness professional for 20 years, Guerra has developed and implemented health promotion programs in worksite, hospital, university, community, and health club settings. Guerra is a certified health education specialist with a master's degree in health promotion management.

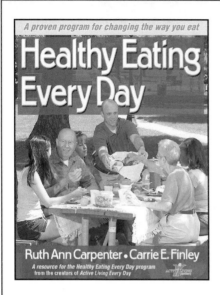
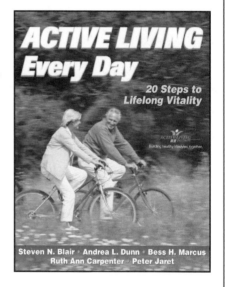